S O U L
RETURN

Integrating Body, Psyche & Spirit

by
Aminah Raheem, Ph.D.

Aslan Publishing
Lower Lake, California
USA

Published by

Aslan Publishing
11270 Clayton Creek Road
PO Box 108
Lower Lake, CA 95457
(800) 275-2606

Library of Congress Cataloging-in-Publication Data:

Raheem, Aminah
    Soul return : integrating body, psyche & spirit / by Aminah
Raheem. — 1st ed.
       p. cm.
    Includes bibliographical references.
    ISBN 0-944031-10-2 : $ 12.95
    1. Whole and part (Psychology) 2. Holism. 3. Transpersonal
psychology. 4. Soul. I. Title.
BF202.R34 1991
150.19—dc20

                                     90-43487
                                         CIP

Cover photograph by John Wimberly
Cover design by Brenda Plowman
Book design by Dawson Church
Printed in USA
SecondEdition

10 9 8 7 6 5 4 3 2

CONTENTS

This book is dedicated to
Muhammad-Subuh Sumohadiwidjojo,
that Great Soul and Bodhisatva who has just soared
from this earth after blessing it with his presence for 87 years.
He gave the original inspiration for this book when he told us
that one day we would discover the psychology of the soul.
He has been my spiritual father and guide for all of this life;
his gifts were and are of unspeakable value.

ACKNOWLEDGMENTS

This book was created out of a tapestry of consciousness woven through myriad interactions through the years with many special individuals—members of my family, teachers, students, colleagues and friends who have inspired, encouraged and supported me throughout the search for understanding.

My children, Paulina, Philip, Rosalind and William Henry, have been a constant source of learning, joy, love and strength. I am forever grateful for their existence. Lauren Stomel, a first-class publications man, my son-in-law and former student, supported the book in many psychological and technical ways. My colleague, Laura Sosnowski, assisted and encouraged me continuously with her love and brilliant skill as a process partner.

The team at Aslan Publishing, Dawson Church, Brenda Plowman and Jenny D'Angelo, have been a writer's dream fulfilled. Their loving support and excellent skills made production of the book especially satisfying. Hal Zina Bennett, my first editor, gave inestimable assistance in understanding, editing, clarifying and shaping the original manuscript. I deeply value his sensitivity, vision and friendship. Without his dedicated support the book would still be in manuscript.

I have been especially fortunate to study and work with master teachers who have all generously shared their knowledge, skill and dedication to excellence: Fritz Smith, originator of Zero Balancing, and author of *Inner Bridges*, whose ongoing research has inspired me constantly; Robert Rasmussen, originator of Regenesis, whose friendship and belief in me have urged me on; June Singer, whose wisdom and deep sisterly friendship have provided a steady light;

Iona Marsaa Teeguarden, originator of Jin Shin Do; Gay Hendricks, co-creator, with Kathlyn Hendricks, of Radiance Breathwork, whose on-target intentions and encouragement have helped me greatly; Harris Clemes, master psycho-therapist, who taught me generously and skillfully; Arnold Mindell, originator of Process Oriented Psychology, whose brilliance, originality, and large heart have given me courage; and countless other fine teachers whose gifts are still with me.

Through the years I have also been blessed with hundreds of extraordinary students who have stimulated, awakened and warmed me with their eager willingness to learn, their creativity and spirit. Finally, thanks to the Transpersonal Integration trainees, a dedicated team, who constantly helped in refining and validating the work.

PROLOGUE

C.G. Jung said that "there is only one striving, namely, the striving after your own being." That thought speaks to my work in a way that is, at one and the same time, simple and profound. My own striving for psycho-spiritual wholeness has been a great gift, and a lense that has given me a fine focus on my work. That work has here been translated into the process which I call "Transpersonal Integration," and it is my hope that it will guide others—individuals as well as therapists and consultants—who are interested in developing the body, the psyche (mind and emotions), and the spiritual nature simultaneously.

Traditionally body, psyche, and spirit nature have been addressed separately: medical and bodywork specialists focus on health of the physical body; psychologists investigate the role of the mind and emotions in behavior; and spiritual teachers attend the transcendent function of the soul. This fragmentation of the whole person has brought about extensive specialization and insight into each of the parts, but has often driven us further away from understanding how they work together. In reality, body, emotions, mind, and soul are not distinctly separate factors within the person. Rather, they constitute an ever-changing complex of forces which interact in extra-ordinarily intricate ways. My own search for wholeness began with separate investigations of these. The spiritual discipline called Subud brought a sense of peace and purpose to my soul, but along with it came a corresponding upheaval in my personality and physical health. I learned that this apparent disorganization in mind and body was understood in many spiritual practices as a normal process of "purification." I was willing to accept this

3

purification to gain spiritual realization, but I wanted to fully understand the process I was going through, if that was possible. This experience led me to seek a deeper understanding of the psychophysical processes involved.

In my study of psychology, I found some clarification for how the mind and emotions operate, and how personality patterns are formed in the process of the person's development. Yet the inner, spiritual process was hardly recognized in this field, and the body was also largely ignored.

As I worked with both adults and adolescents on a psychological level, I began to see that psychological understanding and development often required work with the physical body, a conclusion that has become common among psychologists and bodyworkers who have made important connections between psyche and body. As a result of my realizations, I began to explore the body and its energy systems through the study of a variety of bodywork approaches. Within the Chinese medical model I found a holistic and integrative view of the body, which includes the psyche. I started working with the body through the hands-on technique of acupressure, based on the Chinese model. I found that psychological healing processes were clarified and accelerated by combining bodywork and psychotherapy.

About the same time that I began working with acupressure, I discovered transpersonal psychology, a field that recognizes and respects spiritual development. As a teacher of bodywork, and a doctoral student at the Institute for Transpersonal Psychology, I observed and worked with students who were progressing through a transformation process that involved a combination of psychological, spiritual and body work. Over a period of ten years, during which I worked on myself and with others in a therapeutic practice, an understanding of the whole person began to emerge for me, and finally I received a clear vision of the process I now call "Transpersonal Integration." In the following pages, I present the integrative model as well as some of the possible therapeutic applications that are the basis for this system.

CHAPTER ONE

AN OVERVIEW OF THE WHOLE PERSON

I am that which began;
Out of me the years roll;
Out of me God and man;
I am equal and whole;
God changes, and man,
and the form of them
bodily; I am the soul
—Algernon Charles Swinburne

Fragmentation or Wholeness?

A vision of wholeness was perhaps better understood in ancient times than it is today. Within the Egyptian, Vedic, and Chinese traditions a human being was an indissoluble whole, whose thoughts, emotions and actions issued from total being. But this holistic view of the person, held by ancient peoples and preserved in various esoteric teachings, has today been overshadowed by a rationalistic and scientific tradition.

Although modern scientific methods have produced greater understanding and prediction of the millions of bits and pieces of the human being (including cellular and sub-cellular levels), it has also produced a highly fragmented view of the human experience.

At present some psychologists, holistic health and medical practitioners, and spiritual teachers are trying to fit the pieces back together, and to find therapeutic approaches which will facilitate personal wholeness. Examples of these are: Psychosynthesis (Assagioli); Holonomic Approach (Grof); Radiance Breathwork (Hendricks and Hendricks); Process Oriented Psychology (Mindell); and Integrative Body Therapy (Rosenberg); to name just a few.

In the process of exploring the new wholism, I would like to begin with a fresh look at what are traditionally viewed as the "parts" of the person. In the material presented in this chapter, I will be setting the stage for integrating these parts in a way that takes us one step closer to overcoming the fragmented vision of the human experience. The parts we will examine here are: the soul, the physical body, the mind, and the emotions as they are seen integrated through the factor we call energy.

Soul as an Integrating Factor

My own contribution to a view of wholism begins with an understanding of the spiritual essence or soul, and how it functions as an organizing principle of the whole person.

The concept of the soul as an immaterial principal, essence, or energy which animates life, appears in most philosophical and religious literature from the earliest recorded history, Eastern and Western, yet it is not easily defined. The soul is "the animating and vital principal in man—forming an immaterial entity distinguished from, but temporarily co-existent with, his body." It is the "divine essence" of the whole human being. I see the individual soul as a discrete energy pattern which carries an evolutionary record of its immortal journey. It brings a blueprint for the essential meaning and purpose of the current lifetime, which, in turn, may be part of an evolutionary pattern. The soul is not limited to the attributes of matter.

In this work I distinguish individual soul from Spirit. Spirit is defined as that all-encompassing, creative Order of the Cosmos which is before all beginnings and beyond all endings. Spirit has been called God, the Creator, the Tao, "All That Is." It is seen as the formless all-pervasive energy from which all of creation

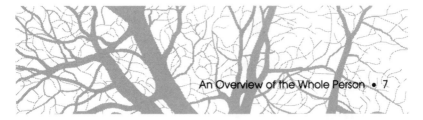

derives, including the individual soul of humankind.

Individual soul originates in, and is permeated by, Spirit, yet it carries a unique expression of its own. The soul is held to be immortal, having existence before and after any given lifetime. At death some part of consciousness from this life travels out of the body with the soul. In esoteric literature this part is called the causal body.

Transpersonal psychology recognizes the existence of the soul and respects its importance as a guiding force, beyond ego, within the whole person. A soul quality has been named by various psychologists. For example, Jung wrote of the Self, Assagioli referred to the higher self, Gurdjieff spoke of essence, and Hendricks, Grof and others speak of the Being. These names are given to distinguish an essential spiritual quality within man and woman which is not mind, not body, not ego nor personality, but which may envelop and influence all of them.

The Physical Body

The physical body is the most concrete form through which the formless soul can manifest. The body is comprised of "the entire material structure and substance of (the) organism." (*American Heritage Dictionary*). The living organism we call the body is composed of some 10–100 trillion cells (*Encyclopedia of Human Histology*, 1984), which organize themselves into eleven physiological systems.

In addition to its function of continuously maintaining an organic form, the body also imprints life experience into its tissues. Various bodywork modalities, distinct from medical approaches aimed at helping organic maintenance, have demonstrated that long-forgotten traumas can be elicited from the body when it is handled or moved in certain ways. These imprintings from experience are understood in psychology as "unconscious material," but it is still not widely known in the field that they are accessible directly through the body. Bodywork has shown that the body is a faithful recorder of personal history. Therefore it is a fruitful ground for understanding and bringing to consciousness those traumas which, according to psychological theory, have shaped personality.

The Emotions

The concept of emotions is not clearly defined despite almost a century of psychological investigation and allusions to emotional experiences in literature and science throughout recorded history.

At the present time in psychology, it is common to make no clear distinctions between mind, or thoughts, and emotions. Jung and others have lumped these together under the term "psyche," although Jung defined the function of feeling as distinct from thinking in his types model. Psychotherapists who work intimately with the psyche, however, can and do make an empirical separation between thought and emotion.

Some contemporary psychologists work primarily with emotion. The focus of their therapeutic approaches is on teaching clients how to regain contact with feelings that have been lost in our primarily rationalistic approach to life. While some psychologists have composed vast catalogues of emotions, others reduce emotion to a basic repertoire of two to five states. Such investigators seem to believe that the release of old traumatic emotion, together with the ability to be aware of emotional states, will bring personal freedom.

There is some evidence that emotional signals are distinct from mental signals in the brain. Penfield, famous neurosurgeon and researcher at McGill University in Montreal, made an effort to demonstrate that emotions, as distinct from thought, are recorded in certain parts of the brain. Similarly, it has been known for several decades that the hypothalamus transmits emotional signals. Other research indicates that emotions can be associated with the limbic system, while thinking processes originate in the cerebral cortices.

I define emotion as "an electrochemical wave phenomenon expressed through the body, involving conscious, visceral, and behavioral changes." This definition allows for the observable phenomenon that an explicit emotion seems to pass through the body and consciousness in a wave-like motion, with a beginning, where awareness is subtle or weak; a middle, where the feeling crests or has full expression; and an end, where the physiological effects in the body settle down toward a state of equilibrium or calm. This perspective suggests a way to work with emotions which honors their valuable expressive capacities without allowing them to take over consciousness. We will be exploring this further in the chapters that follow.

The Mind

In *The Brain Revolution*, (1973) Marilyn Ferguson stated that "No one knows what consciousness is, what mind is. Nor is there any reason to expect blinding illumination from researchers next year or the next decade." Although I generally agree that this is true, I would like to establish a working definition of "mind" as the observed effects of intellectual, unconscious, superconscious and intuitive functions. Such functions combine to effect the complex mental activity that includes storage of bits of information within the organism (probably predominantly within the brain, although this has not been conclusively determined), as well as the organization, retrieval and analysis of that information. Much of this activity can go on with very little physiological arousal, unlike the action of emotions, for example.

A thought may cause an emotion, which in turn can bring about a whole body excitation. On the other hand, thought may persist through much of a day without such physiological effect. Psychologists throughout the past century have devoted much time to the study of this realm and have consequently learned a great deal about it.

The mind-brain operates as a master control over the autonomic nervous system. Research in the last 20 years has demonstrated that the mind can even override the autonomic nervous system. Physiological data now exist to explain what yogis have been demonstrating through the centuries—that heartbeat, oxygen utilization, etc. can be voluntarily controlled. The mind, therefore, commands great potential power over the entire person, according to the refinement of its development. That is, when it holds a broad, relatively accurate data base, and has the developed mental skills to apply that data base, it can become a refined instrument to guide productive life.

Brain research and cognitive development have been emphasized throughout the history of psychology (paralleling modern emphasis on the scientific method of inquiry), which is predominantly mental. There are two broad results of this emphasis: 1) the extensive potential and power of the human mind to collect information, analyze and predict phenomena, and even influence phenomena, has been dramatically demonstrated; and 2) the simultaneous neglect of other parts of the whole human being—body, emotions and spirit—has brought about an unbalanced approach to life. In Western culture, particularly, the educated person tends to be "head-centered," convinced that the solution to human problems lies in the collection of more data, more complex analysis and greater mental understanding.

Clearly, the mind is capable of vast and wonderful accomplishments, contemporary technology being one notable example. However, as an isolated instrument inadequately attuned to the body, emotions and soul of the whole individual, the mind can guide a person (or collectively, a culture) into creations and courses of action that do not serve the whole of the person, a culture, or the environment.

The Parts Make a Whole

These parts intermingle and coalesce within us in extraordinarily complex ways as we develop from birth to adulthood. It is customary in ordinary life to focus our attention on developing one part of ourselves at the expense of the other parts. For example, we may attain great intellectual proficiency while completely neglecting the soul or the body. Or the spiritual seeker may attend exclusively to soul attunement without developing the complimentary mental and emotional foundation to carry the soul's purpose. The athlete or body builder, similarly, may ignore emotional or spiritual promptings, sacrificing them to his/her concern with the body.

Interestingly, the more lopsided we become, concentrating our energies on a single part, the more some other part of us cries out for attention. Signals from neglected parts of the body, mind or emotions will be given—through desires, phobias, hunches, or symptoms—which demand care. And if they are ignored for too long, they will become increasingly insistent, progressing toward self-destructive habits, accidents, or disease.

Thus, even in the midst of our fragmentation something pushes us toward wholism. Jung claimed that we carry "an archetype of wholeness" within us which is always at work to bring us toward fullness and self-realization. Carl Rogers called it the "lead growth shoot" which, like the seemingly fragile but persistent top growth shoot of the pine tree, will keep guiding the organism toward full growth.

Distinguishing Soul From Personality

I distinguish the soul, as the spiritual component of the whole person, from the personality, which is developed through external conditioning.

The study of the personality—its formation, patterns, and influence on daily life—has been the domain of traditional psychology. It is generally accepted in classical psychology that the personality is the person. And that person is seen as the product of parental and environmental influences of the current lifetime. The study of the soul, on the other hand, has been largely contained within religious and spiritual teachings, until the advent of transpersonal psychology, which is attempting to integrate the spiritual nature with the psychological.

In my own work, I see the soul as carrying the essential nature of the self—which includes the evolutionary record and purpose for the current life. I have found that the person develops from the soul center outward, in progressive personality layers that form around it. The personality encapsulates the sum total of accumulated life conditioning which is carried in the body, mind and emotions. It is a creation of the current life and it dissolves at death, whereas the soul is eternal.

Ideally, these two forces—soul and personality—would be integrated and aligned in common purpose, with the personality acting as a vehicle through which the soul might fully manifest its purpose and destiny. This is not always the case, however. The personality is molded in the current life, guided by parents, teachers and institutions who are frequently not attuned to the nature and purpose of the child's soul. More often, the personality of the child is molded by the personal psychologies and common collective values of the time, which may or may not result in a "vehicle that serves its soul." As a result, the personality may actually become an obstruction for the expression of the soul.

A personality is valued according to how well it enables the person to interact with the environment. A severely neurotic or psychotic personality, for example, may be unsuccessful in managing even the most basic tasks of life. It is also true that a personality can function successfully, to all outward appearances, with the person enjoying high levels of achievement in terms of society's values, while not at all satisfying the needs of the soul. All goes well as long as there are not great changes either in the personality or in the social systems that are supporting that personality. But at some critical time, frequently during mid-life, the person may begin to feel that his/her pursuits have been empty. Something else within the person, long neglected, cries out to be heard. At this point, those adaptations to society which have been the source of so much personal satisfaction up to now, may cease to satisfy.

Thanks to the study of psychology, we know a great deal about the structure of the personality and its development. Such knowledge helps us understand the mental/emotional constructs that influence a person's thinking, feeling and behavior. But most of the theories familiar to psychologists do not address the factors of soul and body. So we may work psychologically with the personality and never integrate the essential nature and purpose of the whole person—including all the promptings of the soul and the body, with their seemingly limitless strivings for wholeness. Often the goal of psychotherapy is to make small shifts in the personality so that it may function more successfully within society's structure of values. But this strategy may not be successful for the person whose soul is striving for a different kind of expression or for people who live in a predominantly neurotic or destructive society. As Eric Fromm noted in his analysis of the Nazi society, it was insane to adjust to an insane society.

Energy as an Integrating Factor

What is this single guiding and unifying factor that can bring all the parts into a harmonized whole? Clearly it must interpenetrate all the parts simultaneously and exert an integrating effect. I believe this factor is the flow of energy in the human system. I work through the meridian and chakra energy systems to access and follow the process of the whole person.

Investigation of the human energy system is a recent one in the West. Mesmer postulated the existence of a force he called "animal magnetism"—a force that could heal. Wilhelm Reich's work with "orgone energy" laid a fundamental and profound foundation for understanding bodymind/energy relationships, and his work has been the basis for many bodywork systems in this century. The revolutionary work of Swedish researcher Bjorn Nordenstrom, which postulates an electric circuitry in the body, promises a much greater understanding of energy in the body. But it has virtually gone unnoticed in the field of medicine.

In the East, however, the phenomenon of human energy has been widely recognized and employed therapeutically in empirical practice for thousands of years. In the oldest known documented medical approaches—Ayurvedic (estimated as beginning fifth century B.C.) and Chinese (2698–2599 B.C.)—energy is understood as a primary factor of life, indeed it makes the difference between life and death. The energy systems of the body are just as important as any organic system.

From the Chinese we have a map of human energy flow, charted through some 20 basic pathways (meridians) which are all interconnected. The meridians trace a complete energy circuit within the body every 24 hours. Through several hundred acupoints—windows into the meridians—there is direct access into the meridian energy flow. Similarly, from yogic texts of India, we have descriptions of seven basic energy centers (chakras) which are also interconnected and serve all parts of the body. The energy centers are also found in Chinese theory (Taoism in particular), although they are somewhat different in number and location.

In both systems these energy pathways and centers are correlated with organs and glands in the body, various emotional states, and conditions of consciousness. Energy flow is understood as cutting across all aspects of the whole person—body, mind, emotions and soul. When the energy channels and centers are open—that is, with energy flowing freely and unobstructed through them—the person enjoys a fluid sense of wholeness that includes good physical health, emotional balance, mental clarity and the spiritual well-being which results from being in tune with one's own soul and the spirit of nature. Conversely, if energy flow is obstructed in any one channel or center, corresponding physical, emotional and mental imbalances ensue.

Correlations between energetic conditions of the body and combinations of physical symptoms, emotional, mental and spiritual states are outlined in the traditional texts. During the last ten years there has been significant empirical investigation of how these ancient understandings can be applied to contemporary Western bodies.

The growing use of acupuncture, acupressure and chakra energy has demonstrated that energetic balancing in the body automatically brings about increased well-being, on an emotional level, with an improvement in intellectual function. I have found that the energy systems of the body provide an excellent model of energy for assessing and integrating body, mind, emotions and soul. By paying attention to energy flow we can more easily read just which level is unbalanced and then access it appropriately.

Direct work in the energy systems of the body will automatically and simultaneously affect all other aspects of the body, mind, emotions, and soul. Furthermore, by following leads in these systems we can (1) assess those parts of the individual that most need attention and support; and (2) address those parts with the most appropriate therapeutic tools. Intervention, change or rebalance can be effected according to the natural tolerance of the whole system. Through facilitating and following the natural adjustment of energy flow, we can organically support a person's wholistic growth process with minimal risk. This means that we can move at a pace, and with an energetic power level, that the person can work with harmonically.

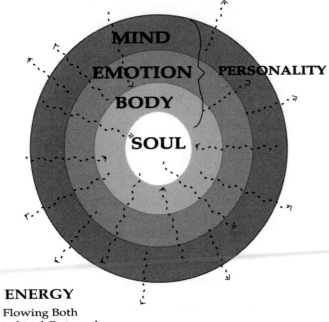

ENERGY
Flowing Both
Inward and Outward,
Integrates the Whole Person

ILLUSTRATION 1

The Path to Personal Integration

The person who wishes to realize his whole self undertakes a journey that will go through many stages—physical, psychological, transpersonal and spiritual. Recovery of the soul from the morass of fragmentation and personal conditioning is not an automatic, nor even "normal" development in life. Rather, it is an extra-ordinary project that requires awareness of every realm of the whole being. It is such an unusual task, in fact, that Gurdjieff taught that it could not be done without the aid of a master teacher. The path will eventually lead beyond social adjustment, beyond successful personality and into transpersonal or spiritual dimensions. The work is wholistic and comprehensive.

Transpersonal Integration seeks to bring about integration of the body, mind and emotions with soul direction. It is designed to work with all stages of the self-realization journey. Physical, psychological and spiritual work are incorporated because all are necessary for this constantly unfolding process.

For example, psychological personality work to extricate a person from the bonds of parental and social programming is a necessary and integral part of the process. When this phase nears completion, the spiritual work of soul direction emerges. Self-realization, or individuation, will require reclaiming the soul and honoring the direction it provides. This stage has been traditionally guided by religious and spiritual disciplines. Indeed, some spiritual practices can activate the soul directly by opening energetic channels through the personality for an influx of divine energy and higher guidance. When spiritual practices are combined with appropriate psychological personality work, as in Transpersonal Integration, self-realization can proceed from within and without simultaneously.

Throughout this journey, the body needs release, adjustment, and stabilization with the process.

Experiencing Wholeness

A condition of wholeness can be described as one in which a person operates from a unified consciousness of body, mind, emotions and soul. As the bonds of conditioning are shed, one begins to gain fuller awareness of a deep, self-directed process that moves toward self-actualization and harmony with the cosmos. As in childhood, one becomes vulnerable again—to oneself, to other people, and to the vast mystery of life itself. The "still small voice within" can once again be heard.

Where one is guided by the transcendent function of the soul and assisted by many freed parts of the personality, individualized purpose can be realized. One responds to life with free thinking, open feelings, and behaviors that are congruent with the needs of bodymind and are in harmony with the truth of the moment. The soul shines through all the layers of the personality. Such a soul-guided person is in tune with the unfolding, evolutionary flow of the Universe because individual purpose is part of that much bigger order in which we are all mysteriously united through spirit.

Moments of wholeness are not as uncommon as one might suppose. All of us have known of "peak experiences"—as Abraham Maslow called them—moments when, in the words of William Butler Yeats, "You cannot tell the dancer from the dance." The person who lives in a continuous state of wholeness is rare, of course. We generally must search spiritual literature for descriptions of yogis or saints who live in a state of "cosmic bliss," and who still function effectively in the day-to-day world.

Maslow defined the self-actualizing person as one who has fulfilled basic survival needs to the extent that he is able to move further into a creative process for realizing all his potential. The human potential movement has been investigating this potential for over a decade, and transpersonal psychology has taken us even closer to an understanding of spiritual or transcendent needs. Clearly we need new models in this Aquarian age for what a human being can actually become, or it would be more correct to say, what a human being already is but needs to reclaim.

I have always been interested in saints and yogis who demonstrated vast possibilities of human potential beyond the mundane and adaptive. I have read their biographies and journals extensively, looking for clues about their strategies. Of course, reading is seldom enough. But fortunately, within the last ten years I have met and worked with enough self-actualized individuals to believe confidently that a new order of human being is completely possible. And I also believe that a relatively small number of such individuals in the world—through free creativity and spiritual inspiration—could provide the leadership to enable us to solve our serious global self-destructive problems.

My individual work, both with myself and with my clients, is aimed at furthering all these possibilities. My dreams and visions still support my faith that we are living in that time promised by the ancient Hebrew scriptures in the Book of Jeremiah:

> *After those days, saith the Lord, I will put my law in their inward parts, and will write it in their hearts; and I will be their God, and they shall be my people. And they shall teach no more every man his neighbor, and every man his brother, saying, know the Lord: for they shall all know me, from the least of them, unto the greatest of them.* (Jeremiah, 31:33)

Summary

Body, mind, emotions and soul together form the whole person. Although these factors are not in actuality separate from one another, since their functions overlap and intermingle, they can nevertheless be described as having recognizable characteristics unto themselves. The soul is a free immortal essence which contains the essential purpose or blueprint for life. Life conditioning is imprinted into the physical body. A personality structure is developed layer upon layer from life conditioning that is particular to the family, society and time of the individual life.

Energy within the human system, flowing through pathways (meridians) and centers (chakras), is proposed as the primary factor which interpenetrates and integrates the body, mind, emotions and soul.

The aim of Transpersonal Integration is to facilitate a true psycho-spiritual transformation in which the client can recover the meaning and purpose of his own soul and integrate it with the personality structure. Methods for this process will be described in the closing chapter of this book.

CHAPTER TWO

THE SOUL FACTOR

The dream is the small hidden door in the deepest and most intimate sanctum of the soul, which opens into that primal cosmic night that was soul long before there was a conscious ego and will be soul far beyond what a conscious ego could ever reach.

C.G. Jung, The Meaning of Psychology for Modern Man, 1934

Soul as Foundation for a Wholistic Model

Though discussions about the existence of soul have been found in nearly every recorded philosophy, we have no scientific basis for its existence. Regardless of the lack of scientific evidence, a clear concept of soul is both possible and necessary for developing a wholistic view of the person.

Our model for this book is that the soul is the vital center, the essence of the whole being. It is unique and immortal. According to my investigation, the soul enters a given lifetime as a highly charged energetic matrix or blueprint which contains complex potentials for life realization and incompletions from before the life. It is the spiritual equivalent of the DNA which carries the genetic code for physical development.

The Soul's Historical Record

In working with hundreds of individuals in a psycho-spiritual way, I have come to believe that the soul is not a "blank slate" when it enters a given lifetime, but rather is a concentrated evolutionary record with a highly individualized meaning and history. This record seems to include experiences, images and symbols that cannot be directly associated with the present life history.

Socrates believed that the soul existed before the body. Prior to its immersion in the body, the soul was endowed with all knowledge. However, when the soul entered its present material form it became stupefied. Socrates believed that the soul could be reawakened and that it could recover its original knowledge. These beliefs were at the foundation of his efforts to stimulate soul-powers through irony and inductive reasoning.

Experiences of pre-life impressions occur frequently in depth psychotherapy, meditation or mystical states, drug experience and other altered states of consciousness. Such material often indicates that human consciousness reaches back in time, to the very roots and evolution of human history. Images, impressions and episodes emerge that could not be explained by present life experiences. Jung defined the deep archetypal consciousness he encountered in many patients as the "collective unconscious," to denote a bank of historical, non-personal information that carried a record of mankind's history. Within that level, we are all connected with a common species heritage.

According to the Eastern view, the soul collects a history, including knowledge, traumatic (or unfinished) experiences, strengths, skills, debts (or karma)—the sum and consequences of many previous lives. During the long evolutionary journey from a soul's infancy to its maturity (which may encompass thousands of years), it accumulates information about life on earth. It carries within itself the record of these past experiences, which can exert influences upon the present life to effect certain achievements or repayments of karmic debts, certain completions and healings.

In my own personal therapy and within the development of some hundreds of clients I have worked with, the incidence of

"past lives material" has been important. Memories have been retrieved from the soul level of consciousness which have no correspondence to history in the present life. Often these "memories" provide keys to present life problems or they reveal limiting patterns which can be resolved, changed, or transformed. Whether a soul record derives from a history of past lives or spiritual essence is a scientific unknown, of course, but its content can nevertheless provide valuable insight and metaphorical guidance for the successful realization of the whole human being.

Links With Universal Spirit

In Chapter One, I differentiated individual soul from the more universal entity I call Spirit. According to most spiritual teachings, the soul originates from Spirit, which is the "all-encompassing, creative order of the Cosmos." Taoist Master Ni Hua-Ching writes in *The Uncharted Voyage Toward the Subtle Light:*

> *The spirit itself is infinite so that it may also appear in personal form. It is free of any definition and it does not need any conceptual doctrine....The Spirit is impersonal energy whereas the soul is personified....At death the personified soul returns to Spirit which carries the root of life forward.*

The individual soul carries within itself the spark or "light" of Universal Spirit. Thus it is permeated with, and attuned to, the great "silent pulse of the universe," which George Leonard describes in *The Silent Pulse:*

> *At the heart of each of us, whatever our imperfections, there exists a silent pulse of perfect rhythm, a complex of wave forms and resonances, which is absolutely individual and unique, and yet which connects us to everything in the universe.*

Since the soul is infused with "all-pervasive stuff of the universe," which also infuses all other souls, it is capable of being one with all others at a spiritual level. Yet paradoxically, the individual soul is unique, comprising an individuality never duplicable. It is an essence or a seed which brings its own pattern to be realized, and that individual pattern is also an integral part of a greater universal pattern. Thus, the individual soul can resonate to the order of the Universal Spirit. Leonard says:

> At each step along the way, every entity is connected to the great web of information that is the universe....Though all the information of the universe is ultimately available "in" each of us, the amount of it we can encode and express—a tiny amount, indeed—is limited by our particular history, culture, language and nervous system.

Tasks of the Soul

In my own experiences with clients, the soul seems to bring two broad tasks to life. They are to:
1) carry out personal destiny, and
2) build the form and context to execute that destiny.

At birth the soul has the information and energy—forming a kind of time-released blueprint—necessary for the execution of individual destiny in the life ahead. Destiny is defined as "a potential for certain actions, realizations, creative expressions or accomplishments in life." For the individual, destiny is the realization of the soul's blueprint. I call this energy/information complex of the soul the "Master Program."

Although the infant expresses the soul, it is by no means equipped to carry out its soul's destiny. Body, mind and emotions as they accumulate life experience will constitute the material through which the soul executes its destiny. "A soul cannot develop and progress without our appropriate body, because it is the physical body that furnishes the material for its development" (Hartmann, quoted in Hall, 1977).

Life becomes a constant balancing process between the soul's push to fulfill its destiny and the pull of the physical world, that is, the environmental and material forms that life takes. The soul, being of Spirit, wants to live in Spirit; the material form in which that spirit exists (body, mind, and emotions) wants to live out

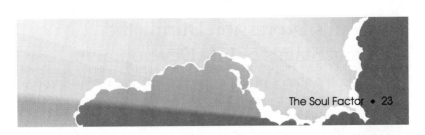

that material form. For example, the soul that is dedicated to a destiny of service to mankind will need to build the physical strength and stamina, the mental understanding and focus, the emotional compassion and the significant connections with people, that will enable it to fulfill its destiny. Yet any one of these skill developments could easily become a dominant preoccupation and distract the person from overall soul purpose. For instance, building a strong body can become a life concentration in itself and can woo the body-builder into the belief that the body comes first and is predominant, to be served by all other parts of the being. Similarly, intellectual development can consume life's attention and direction.

The process of balancing worldly or material achievements against the unfolding of soul destiny might be described as an intricate choreography, always moving toward wholeness:

> *The cross, or whatever other heavy burden the hero carries, is himself, or rather the self, namely his wholeness, which is both God and animal—not merely the empirical man, but the totality of his being which is rooted in his animal-nature, and reaches out beyond the merely human towards the divine. His wholeness implies a tremendous tension of opposites.* (Jung, 1967)

In Western philosophy a duality between soul and matter was first articulated by Plato. Thereafter, traditional Western religious practice emphasized soul to the exclusion or even destruction of the body. Focusing predominantly on spiritual direction and expression, such practices have sometimes obscured the understanding that the material form has been created by and for the soul, entirely for the purpose of carrying out its own needs and purposes. At the opposite pole, those who sought worldly achievement (through reason and science) tended to become attached to and dominated by material forms to the exclusion of the soul's direction.

The Soul's Expression During the Different Stages of Life Development

During the stages of life development from conception to death, the process of balancing spirit and form fluctuates between a dominance of soul and a dominance of bodymind/emotions. In the following sections we will follow the soul's path through these stages.

THE PRENATAL PERIOD

When the soul takes on or creates a physical body, it brings its history and purpose, as described above, into that body or vehicle. It will also take on the genetic complex of the two parents. This genetic coding will influence how the soul's purpose can be realized in form.

The exact time when the soul enters the body is a matter of religious and esoteric speculation. It has been proposed that this union occurs at conception, in the third month of gestation, a year after birth, etc.

Many people undergoing therapy, or through religious and drug experiences, have reported a sense of themselves as "pure being" or "pure soul" during the prenatal period. For example, a man reported being identified with the sperm as it moved up the vaginal channel and then being aware of a burst of light and a sense of completion as it merged with the ovum.

In Eastern cultures it is believed that the soul chooses its parents (and therefore the fetus) according to past connections with them and/or characteristics and conditions for life which the parents can provide. Edith Fiore, past life therapist and author of *You Have Been Here Before*, reported at the Association for Past Life Research and Therapy Conference (Oakland, 1983), that in 2,000 past life regressions she found about 80% of the clients claimed previous connections with parents.

In a therapy session, in an altered state, I experienced this stage of the soul's initial contact for myself. I include a description of that experience as an example of how this revelation can occur:

> *I'm hovering about the fetus. I am in it and yet much bigger than it. In fact, I extend far beyond the body of the mother out into the environment, the consciousness of the father, and into a large,*

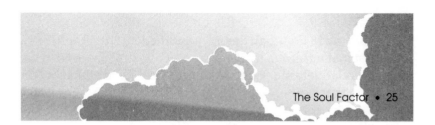

*geographical space around where they live. I am in contact with
my Source. I know what I'm doing. I remember my true home. I
know why I'm taking on physical life now, and I am creating the
body just as I need it to be. I am a creative wave motion, fashion-
ing the energy and substance of the body from the genetic
material of the mother and the father. I am working all the way
into the cells.*

*I am aware of, but not attached to, mother and her condition. My
essence infuses her and influences her but she is not aware of
this. I am not confined at all by the fetus; I extend far beyond it,
to my Source, while still in this dimension. I am free to travel in
a vast space that extends beyond this world. And yet I am always
concentrating on the creation of this body. It's an important
"project." I know already many of the things that will happen to
me in this life coming up. I know the specific tasks I've set for
myself. I want to remember home and the path back to it after
this life is finished. And I can already see how that memory will
become clouded, how I can lose touch with it. I concentrate very
intensely to infuse my body with enough of myself so that it will
always have contact with this knowing, this energy.*

A number of my clients have described similar awareness of
the prenatal period. The soul seems to remain present, gradually
attuning itself to the physical form, yet knowing its existence and
purpose beyond that form. I believe that some of the sense of
oceanic bliss that Freud associated with the gestation period may
have to do with this soul-predominant state, rather than an ideal,
all-nourishing condition provided through the mother's womb.

Throughout the prenatal period and into the birth experience, the soul continues to exert a guiding influence while it is
simultaneously investing itself in form and taking on the corresponding experiences and conditions.

Birth

According to Freudian theory, amplified by Otto Rank, birth is the first major trauma in life. Dramatic physical changes to the fetus in a relatively short period of time may have an impact on the system that can have lasting affects. The soul may or may not be affected by this physical trauma. If the prenatal period has been relatively benign, and the soul is still the predominating influence over the fetus, an infant can flow with and through the uncomfortable physical ordeal of birth with little or no trauma. For example, one of my clients, who got in contact with her own birth experience during an altered state, described it thus:

> *I am entering the phase of birth. I sense its preparation in energy, the body of my mother and my own physical body. I am watching the process of labor contractions as their progressive waves move me through the birth canal. My awareness pervades all elements of the process. I am in my mother's consciousness, know her thoughts and feelings, her physical pain (there is a slight guilt forming about this). I am also aware of pressure—I wouldn't call it pain—on my own physical body. At the same time, most of me is apart from this, observing with interest. If I choose to, I can completely enter into the process at a physical level. This is painful, suffocating, imprisoning, terrifying. But I can withdraw from that identification and I am again a soul, watching a natural and beautiful unfolding of the life process.*

When the physical and emotional conditions of gestation are not life-promoting, the soul may become enmeshed in a survival struggle that drives it deeply into identification with the body. For example, if one or both parents do not want the child, if there are unsuccessful abortion attempts, or if the mother's body is not carrying sufficient life-giving properties (due to inadequate nutrition, disease, or drug saturation), the soul can be aware of its precarious hold on physical life. In fact, the soul can experience rejection before it is ever birthed.

A client experienced the medium of her mother's womb as almost completely toxic. Her mother was a heavy alcohol drinker; she did not want the child and experienced frequent depression. The client described her experience as follows:

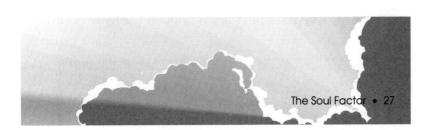

They (the parents) are fighting over me again. Neither of them wants me. Each blames the other. My mother's depression is so heavy that it feels like swimming in a black swamp. I feel drugged. I don't want to come into this environment. Who will support me? Who will teach me how to live?

The experience of birth for such an already burdened soul can be further invalidating and debilitating. As previously mentioned in Fiore's work, it may be that such a soul has karmic reasons to choose rejecting parents. Working out rejection and unworthiness can be part of a soul's destiny.

On the other hand, a soul can remain quite clear at birth and early infancy—charged with its own light, alert and connected with Spirit—especially when it has been welcomed by parents as a worthwhile, loved being.

A sensitive person can experience a condition of purity and clarity hovering about a newborn baby. It is a sweetness, a reminder of Divinity that draws out love, compassion and respect. There is often a sense of heavenly peace in the presence of the newborn. The soul still dominates, and its "light" radiates.

INFANCY AND EARLY CHILDHOOD

As the person develops through infancy and childhood, the process of building the complex form of bodymind/emotions takes over. Programs of conditioning are layered into this complex structure to form the personality. Gradually the personality covers over the soul as most life energy is consumed by simply coping with the environment. Personalities and sub-personalities are formed and somewhere between the ages of 6 to 12, they become generally stronger in expression than the soul.

In general, we train children to fit into existing social structures, roles and behavior patterns. It is rare that the individual soul is even perceived, much less encouraged in its own nature and purpose. As Alice Miller has written in *The Drama of Being a Child*:

> *We arrive in this world full of unlimited potential, wanting to give freely from it, but we find out that this is not what our parents want. They prefer good little boys and girls....For the majority of sensitive people, the true self remains deeply and thoroughly hidden.* (1987)

Even with our parents' molding, however, the soul continues to shine through the layers of conditioning, most often when a child is playing—engaged in spontaneous and free activities that allow her nature to be expressed as she experiments, imagines, and creates in ways that are completely unique, without reference to established methods or codes of behavior.

Some few children are able to retain a high degree of soul contact. Artists, writers, healers and mystics have described childhoods in which they "knew" profound laws of the universe, and felt themselves as being constantly guided from a source larger than themselves. The poet William Blake described his companionship with angels whom he saw and with whom he communicated. Similarly, Mr. A., the healer who is the subject of *Born To Heal* (Montgomery), claimed that from earliest childhood he had a direct contact with "rings of knowledge which surround this planet," which taught him how to heal little animals and even people.

In his autobiography, *The Knee Of Listening*, Da Free John reported a blissful state that he experienced in early childhood which he called "the bright":

> *From my earliest experience of life I have enjoyed a condition that I would call the "bright." As a baby I remember crawling around inquisitively with an incredible sense of joy, light and freedom in the middle of my head that was bathed in energies moving freely down from above, up, around and down through my body and my heart. It was an expanding sphere of joy from the heart. And I was a radiant form, a source of energy, bliss and light.* (1972)

He states that he later lost this state of consciousness and did not regain it until after many years of psycho-spiritual seeking.

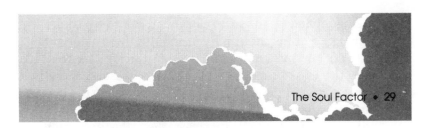

ADOLESCENCE AND ADULTHOOD

By the onset of adolescence, most children are intricately programmed into the cultural complex of their time and place. The "still small voice" of the soul is rarely heard and, when it is, it is usually discarded as fantasy or nonsense. For example, when I worked with late adolescents, I found that they often received deep soul promptings through dreams or visionary experiences. These numinous events seemed to contain valuable guidance for direction in their lives, but usually they were discounted by the dreamers and their peers as fantasy. By contrast, in American Indian culture such experiences are valued as clear messages of life purpose, especially when they appear during puberty.

Conditioning continues at an intense rate through adolescence, early adulthood and into adulthood as a person is being prepared through school and work experience to assume his/her station as a useful citizen. Through these phases of development the personality develops and by adulthood has generally become a fairly fixed structure of patterns. This structure is absolutely necessary and valuable for productive social life; ego and sub-personalities must be built. Cultural conditioning is essential to cultural expression.

When an individual reaches the peak of physical, emotional and mental power during midlife, he may have become so invested in those powers of the body, mind and emotions and their corresponding worldly achievements, however, that the soul is completely forgotten. In such a case, the balance between the soul destiny and worldly personality is lost.

Through the progressive phases of life, then, there is a general tendency for personality to overshadow the soul. An analogy of a master who has been overcome by his pupils helps illustrate this phenomenon: The pupils may take charge of the classroom, write their own lessons, set recess time, and even call school off altogether, while the master, who is eminently qualified to guide their intelligent and healthy development, is tied up under the desk with a gag in his mouth. Even though the master is temporarily out of commission, he still lives and, in fact, his presence influences the classroom. As long as he is present, there is a chance that some bright pupil might decide to untie the master, help him to his feet and allow him to restore order.

The Soul always *lives*. Its *presence* affects the whole person, even when it is willfully ignored. It exerts an unconscious influence throughout life, and will sometimes move into circumstances, relationships, or opportunities that will serve it but which the ego and the personality do not want. They may perceive such out-of-pattern events as threatening to them, which indeed they may be. Ego will fight for dominance. Yet, the soul will continue to prompt the person until there is no more possibility for the fulfillment of destiny, (at which point, it can choose to withdraw and bring the life to a close). It is fortunate for the whole person when ego loses the battle and soul is able to nudge development on toward its actual purpose.

This process was brought to my awareness in a most dramatic way one time as I was working with a 50-year-old woman who was mysteriously ill. She had a progressive paralysis for which medical doctors could find no physiological cause. The paralysis affected her left side and she was rapidly losing her power of speech. A few years before she had suffered a painful separation from her fiancé, which dashed her hope and expectation of marriage and left her in the home of her aging and ailing father, for whom she had already been caring for many years.

At the time I worked with this woman she was in a nursing home. I was asked to work on her body and assess whether I thought acupressure could help her. As I was working with her, I became aware of a strong presence on the other side of the room. I turned my attention to it and "saw" or "felt" the woman's "double." I perceived the double as her soul, observing me working on her body.

My response was one of indignation. Mentally I said to her soul, "Get back over here into your body. It needs you. What are you doing way over there?" The soul's reply was just as startling: "She (the personality) isn't doing anything with her life. She has given up and there is nothing more I can do with her."

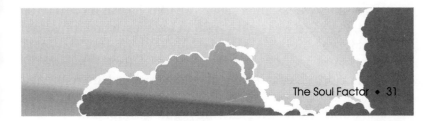

When the soul becomes so covered over by conditioning that it cannot shine through, when personality completely dominates, a "darkness" develops within the person, characterized by mental or emotional dullness, physical deterioration, accidents, depression, or "bad luck." Such a person seems asleep or unconscious while walking around; she has gotten off her own soul path. A return to the soul may come through conscious transformation processes or through great shock, which temporarily dislodges personality structure.

On the other hand, the person who follows her own soul and uses the vehicle of personality to execute its purpose, will become "lighter" through life. There will be a sense of flowing easily from one moment to the next, as though she were in a beautifully choreographed dance which she had thoroughly mastered.

The free, expansive soul energy can dance through the whole person, bringing creativity, spontaneity and vitality throughout mind, body and emotions. And since such a person is on course, integrated with her own Tao, she can experience strength, tranquility and certainty from within herself.

Individuation and Soul Purpose

Jung believed that the final and most important task of life was individuation—an unfolding process in which a person would come fully into his own self, or soul, and live out its purpose. He believed that this phase of development could only be accomplished in the second half of life, when there was enough maturity, experience of life, and awareness of the presence of death to urge the soul forward. True to his lifelong commitment to explore and verify his psychological postulations within himself, he followed his own individuation process to the end. We have a lucid and fascinating account of this in Jung's *Memories, Dreams and Reflections* (1961).

When Jung was last interviewed on film, he was more than 80 years old, yet there was a clear light in his eyes, emanating from his face. He was "light" in feeling—laughing, vital and engaged. There was no sense of his spirit dulling or deteriorating; on the contrary, he projected a feeling of a flame rising. I am reminded also of Mother Teresa. A light shines far out beyond her small physical frame and her smile literally radiates hope and blessing.

So it is within the whole person who honors the meaning and purpose of soul. As the physical body ages, the soul comes fully forward and finally dominates, as it did in infancy. In the latter stages of life, the person can feel the integrity and satisfaction of a life that has fulfilled its purpose, and a peacefulness about going on through death into the next dimension.

Return to the Soul

The process of individuation requires a return to the deep central meaning of the soul. It is a subtle and complex process that usually unfolds over a lifetime. It is curious, in a way, that we should travel so far from ourselves, out into the world, to weave the intricate adaptive structure of the personality only to find eventually that, having lost ourselves in the morass, we need to find ourselves again by coming back to center, where we began— to that innermost flame of our own being. The return can be a fascinating and creative journey. It can be demanding and uncomfortable. But the reward is to reclaim the joy and purposefulness that inherently belong to us.

A client who had been sincerely working to dismantle the bindings of conditioning had the following dream, which metaphorically describes the gradual uncovering of the Self:

*I saw myself as inside my skin and my skin and outer muscles had been stretched very tight by a set of aluminum things like jacks pushing outward, making my exterior very tight and rigid, to form a defensive shell. Working from the inside, I was very carefully undoing mechanisms one at a time, folding them up so that gradually my outer shell was closer and closer to me. Finally it became soft, pliable and even loose in places before its natural elasticity could re-form it to conform **to my actual contours**. This process was hard work, involving hard physical effort to loosen and turn the mechanisms.*

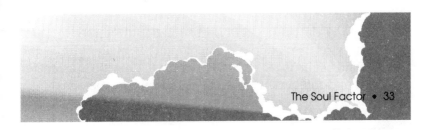

This client's "defensive shell," built to cope with threatening influences throughout her life, was in fact embedded into her body so that her musculature was very tight and rigid when she began therapy. But as her body, mind and emotions began to release, she could sense underneath them the "soft, pliable" nature of her own "actual contours," her own soul identity.

Sometimes the process of uncovering the Self requires assistance. Although the soul always contains all the information it needs to complete its purpose, that information may not be readily accessible because it is too deeply armored by the rigid personality structure. Many growth techniques of the new age, including therapy, spiritual work with a master, meditation, group trainings that preserve individual integrity, and the like, can help. Transpersonal Integration can help people reach the soul level at the earliest appropriate opportunity in the psychological work and so gain access to the wisdom contained in the soul, using that wisdom for further individuation of the Self.

Through the spiritual practice of the Subud *latihan*—a nondenominational spiritual exercise from within—I have witnessed the soul coming alive at the center. Somehow the high intensity energy of the latihan penetrates to the essence of a person and activates it. The soul then gradually begins to radiate out through the personality. This process, usually referred to as "purification," can be disruptive and threatening to the ego, which is comfortable in its personality structure. Gurdjieff taught that such growth of the "being" (soul) from inside was the most important task of life. Any practice which stimulates and supports the actual individual soul can provide the much needed soul-food that makes individuation possible.

Generally it is thought that the Self only communicates indirectly, through profound dreams, visions or other unconscious processes. I have found that it is possible to activate conscious contact with the soul. In fact, the first and most important requirement of a modern man or woman in search of the soul is to recognize the truth and divinity of the soul's presence. Once this truth is realized, and a stable contact is made with it, the person can begin to access that deep wisdom of the Master Program and integrate it into life direction. The personality is then gradually released and reorganized to serve soul direction.

Energy and the Soul

What is the energy of the soul? Or, is soul pure energy? Clearly we have yet to answer these questions scientifically. What we do know raises more questions than answers. For example, Burr was able to detect and measure an organizing energy field surrounding the fetus. Sheldrake postulates that there is a morphic field around organisms that records and transmits information. Could it be that the soul carries its record into life through its own distinct energy field? Most religions claim that something endures after the death of the body. Could this something be an energy field altered and added to by life? If the soul is an energy field, then it would permeate the whole person—body, mind, and emotions—throughout life, and it could provide a continuous influence at the sub-atomic level, where energy becomes matter. This speculation could provide one way of explaining the all-pervasive nature of the soul.

Another speculation about the soul and energy has to do with the factor of light. Throughout mystic literature, there is reference to the "light" of the soul which shines through as a result of spiritual practice. The Chinese esoteric classic, *The Secret Of The Golden Flower*, gives a fascinating instruction to the mystical seeker:

> *When the light circulates, the energies of the whole body appear before its throne....Therefore, you only have to make the light circulate; that is the deepest and most wonderful secret.*
> (Wilhelm, 1962)

If the soul is light, making that light circulate would infuse the whole being with soul direction. One of my clients told me of a near-death experience she had while being driven to a hospital in an ambulance. She couldn't see or feel and could barely hear. Yet she saw a light in her heart and knew that it was important to keep it there—which she found she could do by concentrating

on it! She felt that the flashlight the paramedic occasionally shined at her was helpful in reminding her to keep the light in her heart.

In the last several years I have become increasingly interested in this experience of light. When it occurs in my work with clients there are always attendant healings, visions, transcendent insights and release from mundane tangles of life. Though there is no proof of its relationship to the soul, I believe that it accompanies soul realization.

I discussed energy and light with astrophysicist Arthur Toor who explained: "Light (and gravitrons) are the only energy that is independent of matter. That is, light is generated from matter but once produced, it goes free, is independent of its originating source and then it can go straight and true." (All other energy remains intimately connected with matter which generates it.)

Could it be that the soul, as light, generates itself through the matter of the body, and then, upon completion of its task through that matter, can "go free, straight, and true"?

Summary

In this chapter I have described the soul as the immortal essence of the whole human being. It is aligned with the all-encompassing Universal Spirit which is its source. I have postulated that the personified soul carries a record of its previous evolutionary journey (which may include past lives) that can affect present life. Further, I assert that present life destiny of the soul is carried within it as the Master Program.

Tasks of the soul were posited as: 1) the completion of destiny, and 2) the construction of an appropriate form through body, mind and emotions to carry out that destiny. The soul's expression was described in the stages of development from birth through adulthood. Finally, the energy aspect of the soul was explored.

CHAPTER THREE

THE BODY

*I believe that the human body is
an outrageously ingenious demonstration
of the power of consciousness to turn energy into matter
and matter into energy.*

Brugh Joy, JOY'S WAY

The Body Defined

The body is the ***organized physical substance*** of the person, including everything from sub-atomic particles to intricately interwoven organic systems, and is comprised of some 10–100 trillion cells. These cells differentiate themselves into numerous complex systems such as skeletal, muscular, circulatory, respiratory, digestive, nervous, endocrine, sensory, reproductive, skin and urogenital. This entire complex structure originates from a single egg, of the mother, and one sperm cell, from the father, which become the fetus. The original union will eventually form a complete human body system, which will continue to develop and/or change until death.

Medicine and the health sciences address diseases, malfunctions, and the general health of the body's organic functions—and massive information has been collected in these fields. The information collected about the relationships between mind, emotions and the physical structures and functions has been miniscule by comparison. In this book we will be focusing on these latter interrelationships as they can be brought to light in serving the development of the whole being.

The Body as a Record of Life

Like an extraordinarily complex recording instrument, the body registers every significant event of life. It is a walking history of our lives. This is a bold statement to make, yet in the field of bodywork there is considerable evidence that experiences of life are stored in the body. Practitioners of bodywork modalities such as Rolfing, Bioenergetics, the Alexander Technique, Rosen work, Jin Shin Do acupressure, Zero Balancing, and acupuncture are familiar with the phenomenon of memories stored in the body rising into consciousness from hands-on stimulation. It is a common assumption among such practitioners that old stored traumatic patterns within the body must be released, or "cleared," before a person is able to express and function at his physical and psychological potentials.

Patterns of Body Armor

Reich discovered that the body is "armored" by the contraction of muscles and fascia and the blocking of energy flow, in response to threatening events. Traumatic experiences are incorporated into the body as patterns of armor, where they stay until released. He says:

> *Nearly everyone by maturity has developed not only a few—or many—neurotic traits, but a way of standing, looking, holding the mouth and jaw, speaking, breathing and holding up the chest and perhaps pulling in the pelvis, that are characteristic and set—if not rigid and largely unyielding. These visible, analyzable physical manifestations constitute the outward signs of character armor; they and the inner muscular tensions [are] the character or muscular armoring.* (Reich, *Character Armor*, 1949)

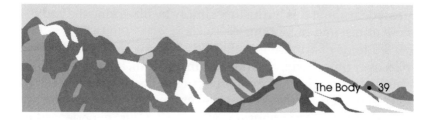

A child falls from his tricycle and in the process suffers the painful experience of a bruised thigh combined with the disappointment or even fear of not being immediately found and comforted by a parent. This complex response is recorded in the body and is stored as information that may guide his actions, thoughts and feelings about climbing onto the tricycle again. All this is translated into muscular responses in the child's body. What began as a simple accident in childhood can thus lead to an uneven gait in the man.

As they grow and develop, from conception to physical maturity, our bodies respond to environmental stimuli, and these responses are imprinted in ways that create a lasting record in the various tissues of the body, and even within the energy system. This gradual accumulation of both pleasurable and painful experience, is imprinted as a complex network of interlocking armor patterns which I have related to the formation of layers of the personality. These patterns guide our body's response at an unconscious level.

The body usually keeps the growing record of life experiences at an unconscious level. For example, the child who fell from the tricycle may be more sensitive to pain or movement on the part of his body where he suffered the original wound. Because of this, he may favor or protect this part of his body; as he does so the neuromuscular pattern established in the original fall is reinforced. What often happens is that a rigid pattern is established that leads to a physical imbalance; the physical imbalance dictates a behavioral response that limits movement and can actually invite further accidents to that area of the body. These rigidities constitute the person's "armor."

Adult bodies are armored with a complex neuromuscular weaving, fashioned from the unique "warps and woofs" of each individual's life experiences. Astute body therapists can read a great deal about this life history simply by observing the body—both at rest and in motion.

Patterns of armoring in the body become increasingly complex over time. Early, or "root" traumas (birth, infancy and early childhood), establish primal programs at the deepest levels that tend to perpetuate themselves in ever more complex and deeply imbedded layers of armoring. A body therapist experienced in releasing this armoring will usually encounter these layers by working from the surface areas to deeper and deeper structures, or from the most recent to the oldest experiences. Depth psychotherapy traditionally progresses in a similar release pattern—from the most recent to the oldest or most regressed material.

Body Armor Related to Personality Layers

As we have seen in Chapter Two, the soul carries the essential meaning and purpose for a lifetime. I have named the deepest, most inviolate level of a person the "Master Program," to denote the soul as the rightful master of the whole human being.

The Master Program holds the true nature of the person, and provides guidance for its realization that is independent from conditioning. For example, the Master Program could carry a broad purpose or "mission," such as service to mankind, or it could carry the program for a narrow, highly specific purpose, such as the discovery and definition of a particular natural law.

Development in form—that is, within body, mind, and emotions—comes about through life experience. Layers of personality begin to build up from environmental conditioning around the soul and Master Program, and it has been my experience that these layers roughly correspond to levels of armoring in the body. Accordingly, I have named these successive levels beyond the soul and the Master Program—the core, the metaprogram, the personality body, and the persona. As armor and personality patterns are "set" into the body, they may limit the free expression of the Master Program. In the following section, personality layers will be described as they form from the soul-center outward.

The Core

The "core" of the person is that soft, vulnerable, innocent body consciousness of the infant that is not yet protected by defense structures. It is very close to the soul and the Master

Program, which still shine through it. The core carries a genetic imprint, that is, the ancestral identifications that come with the body. It also holds "collective unconscious" material—historical imprintings of the human condition which affect all of humanity.

This level of being holds the basic "mythos" of the person, which includes the most primal patterns recorded in body, emotions, and elementary mental processes taken on by the infant. For example, a person who was warmly welcomed, affectionately handled and protected as an infant will most likely carry an unconscious life-affirming message of warmth and safety at the core of his feelings and body. Conversely, the person who endured severe birth trauma or who was abused or neglected in infancy can carry a feeling of insecurity and fear at the core, which translates as a life-negating message.

This level can also include prenatal imprints and the experience of birth. When such experiences are traumatic they can leave formative influences which affect the rest of life in limiting ways.

In actual physical experience the womb medium is not all that comfortable; the fetus is often cramped into uneasy positions. It is subject to the mother's emotional moods. It senses the vibrations of any harsh sounds or untoward physical strains in the mother's body, such as falling, intercourse, etc. Severe trauma can occur during this period.

One client reexperienced a prenatal condition that formed the basis of her lifelong sense of unworthiness. In one therapy session she gained conscious contact with her own prenatal period through regression and attunement with her soul level of consciousness. She reported the following experience:

> *It's very uncomfortable in here. I feel that my very existence is threatened. I'm all squinched over to one side. I can't spread out in the womb because there is a dark area here that is very life-threatening. It's like a big scratch through the womb. I don't*

want to touch there....Oh, my God! I see what it is! Mother had an abortion before I was conceived. She didn't want a baby because she was unmarried and knew her parents would be horrified by unwed pregnancy. Against her wishes she went through with the abortion. I see that this scratch on her womb is the left-over effect of violent intention. I can't trust this place. I can't trust love! She wants me, I feel it, but she wanted the other baby also and that didn't stop her from destroying it.

In a conscious review of this session, the client realized that she had always mistrusted love, even from her overtly loving parents. She refused to ask them for anything from earliest life, even food; she would not cry when hungry. Unconsciously she feared that any demands she would make for life could be answered with extinction.

This particular client carried with her a sense of unworthiness at the deepest unconscious level. Fear was embedded in the physical core until her therapy experience released the trauma into consciousness, where she could evaluate it rationally. She realized that the original abortion was not a rejection of her soul. Over the next few months her attitude of mistrust, which up until that moment had been literally a visceral part of her entire life, began to dissipate. She was able to re-evaluate and take in the true love and caring that her parents had always had for her.

Our relation to our cosmic mother closely parallels that to our physical mother. In that first connection is the seed of all later expectations and fulfillments. If, in the uterus and early extrauterine environment, we were poorly nourished, we will find it emotionally difficult to receive any energies....We will be untrusting, unable to open ourselves to the available nourishment around us. (Kurtz and Prestera, *The Body Speaks*, 1976)

Birth trauma also falls within the core structure. The intense physical pressure, conversion from intrauterine to extrauterine environment, and the pain of the first breath, are all dramatic impacts on the vulnerable physical body. All of these together can cause an organic anxiety reaction in the newborn. In traditional psychology, the primal anxiety is held to be the prototype of all neurotic anxiety. Even a strong traumatic birth trauma, however, can be overridden by the power of the soul.

During the long developmental period that leads to adulthood,

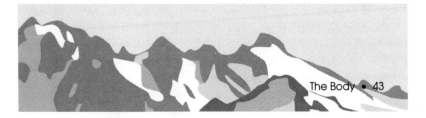

the core imprinting is usually buried beneath many layers of personality and defense structures. Adults are not often vulnerable, innocent, or close to essence as they were in early childhood. In therapy, especially that involving bodywork, or in spiritual growth, a person may reach back into the core of his own vital being and touch the first formative imprints after many more recent issues have been peeled away.

The Metaprogram

The first complex layer of personality begins in infancy and develops through childhood. It is distinguished from the core by its more intricate, and accessible structure. It has been called the "primal" realm of consciousness by Janov, the "metaprogram" by Bandler and Grinder, and the "life position" by Harris. I will refer to it here as the metaprogram.

The metaprogram is composed of early physical, emotional, and some mental imprintings that are stored in the body. Specifically, these imprints can form permanent (unless and until they are changed) biochemical and electrical codes within the hypothalamus and nervous system that can be reactivated by similar stimuli later in life. The metaprogram is therefore deep, forming the primary unconscious material. Since defense mechanisms are not yet firmly in place when it forms, the metaprogram is believed to be nearly indelible. Introjected directives from significant others, traumatic experiences—especially when physical pain is joined with emotional distress—dramatic events, and scripts taken on from others etch their patterns into the unconscious. Fundamental belief systems, from the family and other significant persons or institutions, are also striated throughout the metaprogram.

Examples of metaprogram directives are: a nonverbal script taken on from the family's mode of operation, such as "life is always difficult"; an introjected declaration from mother's continuous criticism, "you are just plain slow," or "you can't get along with your brother"; or a conscious or unconscious decision based on family experience which says "since I can never seem to please them no matter what I do, I might as well get their attention through outrageous behavior."

The metaprogram acts as a powerful matrix program that exerts a strong influence on behavior, thinking, and feeling throughout life. Its primal directives will stay in place, principally within the unconscious, until they are brought into consciousness (the usual work of psychotherapy). This layer forms the skeleton or "deep structure" of the personality. It is the structure which led Freud to postulate that the principle formation of character is established by age six. Most subsequent constructions of the personality will be rooted in this level. Kubie has said that once this layer is established "it becomes the affective position to which that individual will tend to return automatically for the rest of his days. This in turn may constitute either the major safeguard or the major vulnerability of his life" (Kubie, 1958).

Whenever the events leading up to the development of this layer have been painful, a person may spend his entire life defending himself against reexperiencing that pain. He will use conscious, pre-conscious, and unconscious devices whose aim it is to avoid this pain-filled central position.

One of the most fascinating and therapeutically valuable directives that can emanate from this metaprogram level (and also including core and soul level material) is the personal myth, first recognized by Jung and later pursued by a number of Jungians, especially Zurich Jungian analyst Arnold Mindell. The personal myth can come from an early, recurring dream, or from characters or motifs that were prominent in early fantasy. Favorite heroes, heroines, fairy tales, or an early indelible experience often draw the child's mind into a story which can become his/her own mythic directive. This myth can recur over and over, and can propel a person as a kind of inexorable script throughout life. The myth can be positive (heroic) or negative and self-defeating. If it is brought to consciousness through therapy or deep introspection, it can be transformed and redeemed as a central, vitalizing directive, and a very positive force in the person's life. (See Mindell, *Dreambody*.)

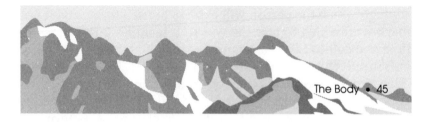

The Personality Body

The principal body of the complex personality is constructed from and around the metaprogram. As the child encounters hundreds of events and influences through all the stages of development into adulthood, intricate personality patterns are formed. The personality will include ego structure, defense systems, a repertoire of roles and sub-personalities. Stone claims that the personality is primarily the many sub-personalities which form during development. Most of these constructions will link back into roots in the metaprogram. For example, the child whose metaprogram contains a message that he is slow will tend to manifest that message in his/her behavior and collect many experiences to verify it. The child who learned that he could not depend on his family to protect him will gravitate toward relationships that are non-protective. On the other hand, early trust in others promotes trusting relationships in later life.

The body of the personality is that part of the person we think of when we say that we "know" a person. It is comprised of certain behavior patterns, certain belief systems, personal opinions, and recurring defense mechanisms. We describe the person we "know" according to some of the many factors which are presented through the personality.

By early adulthood the principal features of the personality are in place. Generally this composite structure will change only through minor reorganizations and refinements through life. Traditional psychotherapy deals principally with this level of the person.

The Persona

The final layer of the personality, the persona, is like a veneer over the entire superstructure. It is the polish or refinement through which the person will express himself to society. It is a mask with which to face the world. It includes adaptations to time and culture, such as manners and ethics, fashion in dress, fads in speech and ways of being in the world. The persona will often be expressed in the form of a role or character type such as "the nice boy," "the bully," "the good little girl," etc. Sometimes a person confuses this veneer with his real self and, in turn, his friends and acquaintances will mistakenly assume that the persona is who that person really is. In reality, an attractive, well-mannered, efficiently organized persona may mask a frightened, resentful, chaotic interior personality which only shows when the person is uncontrollably vulnerable—as in serious illness, drunkenness or shock.

Root Traumas and Neurotic Patterns

Major formative experiences—pleasurable or painful, empowering or defeating—are imbedded into the body throughout development. Such imprints create foundation structures for the personality layers. Positive imprints promote strong personality foundations that can aid the Self in actualizing. On the other hand, some negative experiences can act as root traumas that have a defeating affect on the Self and personality.

The idea of a "root trauma," that is, a profound wound which can shape all subsequent development, was first recognized by Freud. He found that a particularly painful event in early childhood could be buried in the unconscious (and thereby be unavailable to the consciousness) from where it would exert a powerful influence. Barker calls these experiences "critical hurts," and says they are the starting points of neurosis:

> *Occurring usually within the formative periods of growth, hurts are crucial when the individual's instinctive nature, the feeling of himself, his sense of continuity, his image of himself, or essential values of his life have been damaged. I have found that such damage is to be looked for at a juncture where ego consciousness emerges from the instinctual matrix (core is my word); this may occur at any budding phases. Such a buried wound in the personality results in blocking the continuity of the flow of psychic energy within the stem of the personality up*

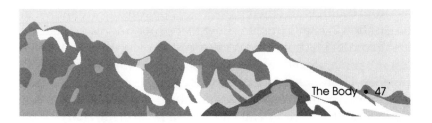

through all subsequent turnings of the spiral growth. (Barker, *Healing in Depth*, 1972)

I have found that root traumas can be imbedded in all layers of the personality (and body), and especially in the metaprogram. A root trauma encapsulates the powerful energy of its original impact. And it requires a tremendous and constant amount of energy to keep it buried. It also acts as a magnetic focus around which subsequent similar traumas (knots) can develop. The root and its related knots reinforce each other as deeply ingrained neurotic patterns.

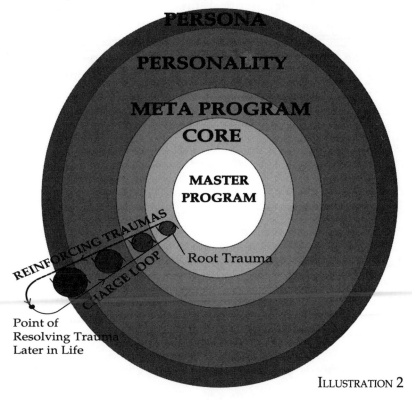

ILLUSTRATION 2

Root traumas and their patterns of relationship are shown in Illustration 2. I have tried to show that a root trauma embedded in the core level attracts and creates traumas with the same theme (for example, abandonment) in subsequent layers of the personality. The root's charge of psychic energy is reinforced by each new trauma, which also creates additional charges of its own that feed back into the root. Thus we have a reinforcing charge loop embedded in the body, which, in my experience, does not release until the root energy is discharged from the body. Further, root traumas can happen in any part of the person—emotional, physical, mental or in combination (as in fact they usually do)—but most will be recorded directly into the body, where their blocked energy is held.

A root trauma can be penetrated, brought to consciousness, and healed, particularly when it is contacted in the body. This action can "pull the plug" on the power of the root trauma in the personality and often start a dismantling process of its structure, as well as all the other knots that draw meaning from it. In my experience, searching out critical hurts is a much more penetrating and efficient way of healing neurosis than analysis at the personality level. A corollary in Oriental medicine is that the adept physician tries to track down the cause or the root of illness, rather than being content to only relieve the symptoms.

Root traumas most often occur in early childhood, as most commonly recognized in psychoanalysis. Recent research shows that root traumas can even occur in the prenatal period. A difficult birth can imprint such a trauma. Once in a while, a very severe trauma, such as severe illness, death of a significant other, etc., can become a root trauma at a later age.

The heavily armored body is also the most highly defended. Such a person has usually become inured to common discomforts, numb to common pain, and also limited in his/her range of physical and emotional response. The heavily armored body can become so insensitive that it no longer heeds pain signals that are so necessary to its own health maintenance. Such a body is more like a programmed machine than the infinitely sensitive, responsive, and intelligent organism that it is capable of being. It responds to the present through built-in patterns shaped by past trauma.

The armored person's habits of protecting and defending

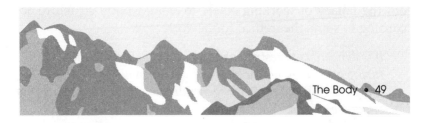

take precedence over his/her capacity to fully experience life. Further, his life direction comes almost exclusively from the ingrained personality structure and the constant avoidance of pain.

I believe, also, that the burden of accumulated past trauma and self-defeating patterns in the body can cause degenerative disease, accidents, and depression in the aging body. It has always fascinated me that old yogis and people who work at maintaining vitality and freedom in their bodies (through exercise, bodywork or some kinds of active physical labor) often reach advanced age in a healthy and vital state. It seems to me that constant physical practice serves to release old trauma from the body, enabling it to respond with strength to current challenges of disease or stress.

Releasing Body Armor

Body armor can be released through appropriate bodywork. In fact, this is the aim of most sophisticated bodywork which is designed to "unhinge" armor patterns in explicit progressions. As such work progresses, the traumas associated with the armoring, as well as related personality factors, are exposed.

> *As imprints are removed from the energy body recollections of past events associated with the original injury often take place. Imprinting of vibration in the body is one basis for the phenomenon of muscle memory.* (Smith, *Inner Bridges*, 1986)

Ideally, armor would be released in layers, from the outer surface to the deep and inner tissue, and the related psychological material would be "processed" along the way. Ideally the integrity and unity of the bodymind/ emotions/ soul would be respected at every step in the process.

In *Working With the Dreaming Body*, Arnold Mindell points

out the fallacy of working solely to change body structure according to some theoretical framework:

> *It is dangerous to restructure people simply because the restructuring goes along with a physical ideal or some theory of health. The term 'normal' cannot be generalized. Each individual has his or her own norm. Process is a matter of what the Chinese call Tao. Timing a change in the body is not up to the therapist, but rather up to the person's body indications.*

Similarly, in psychotherapy, if the personality is explored only through thinking and emotions (analysis) without attendant body release of the neuromuscular layers that keep them in place, there can never be full or permanent release from the armoring. Neurotic patterns are bound into the body, and they tend to come back, particularly under stress. However, when bodywork is combined with corresponding psychological processing, personality patterns can gradually let go and make way for the emergence, once again, of the soul's Master Program.

Body Parts, Energy Pathways, And Related Psychological Material

Now that we have an overview of how the body stores patterns of personality development, it can be useful to learn what kinds of issues tend to collect in which body parts. The remainder of this chapter is a kind of orientation manual on the categories of psychological material that are commonly associated with specific body segments. The information is taken from my experience with hundreds of students and clients and from the growing body of bodywork literature that addresses these correspondences. It can be useful in giving us clues about psychological possibilities as we work with explicit body parts. In the final analysis it is most important in Transpersonal Integration to follow the actual organic process of body releasing, as in Process Oriented Psychology (Mindell, 1985, 1986), and not to get locked into any particular interpretation of content. However, the traditional experience of specific psychophysical correspondences helps to sharpen our awareness.

A number of body maps from established bodywork modalities are used here to illustrate correlations between body

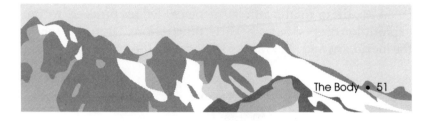

parts and psychological content. The most important of these, in my experience, are the ancient energy maps of meridians and chakras, as introduced in Chapter One, since it is through energy that the body is integrated and unified. (See Illustrations 3–6.) Thus, each of the body parts or segments will be defined primarily through their energy correspondences. Transpersonal Integration is designed to read the body, and to correct imbalances, principally through the energy matrix.

It is essential to bear in mind that all parts of the body are interconnected—physiologically and energetically. What affects one part will eventually influence others, especially within the energy system. For example, there are eight overall supervisory energy channels (the eight "extraordinary meridians") which directly connect all meridians and parts of the body and work continuously to preserve integrity and balance.

In addition to the overall balancing functions of the extraordinary meridians, the following principles of Traditional Chinese Medicine apply when we work energetically in the body:

1. Energy (Qi or chi) flows continuously in a 24-hour circuit within the entire body/consciousness. Energy, therefore, cannot be separated into isolated parts, although its specific pathways (meridians) can be used to identify patterns of imbalance.

2. As above, so below: Imbalances or distortions in upper regions of the body (cervical spine, chest, head, etc.) will be reflected in corresponding imbalances in the lower regions (pelvis, legs or feet), and vice versa. (It is well known by chiropractors and osteopaths that cervical spine problems will reflect in the sacrum.)

3. As in the front, so behind: Imbalances or hurts in the front of the body will often be reflected in a corresponding area straight through to the back, and vice versa.

With these qualifications in place, let us proceed to our exploration of specific body parts. Illustrations 3 through 9 show the meridians and chakras associated with these body segments.

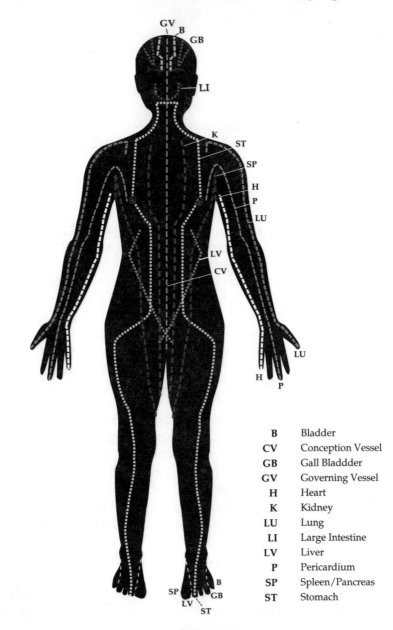

B	Bladder
CV	Conception Vessel
GB	Gall Bladdder
GV	Governing Vessel
H	Heart
K	Kidney
LU	Lung
LI	Large Intestine
LV	Liver
P	Pericardium
SP	Spleen/Pancreas
ST	Stomach

ILLUSTRATION 3: FRONT MERIDIANS

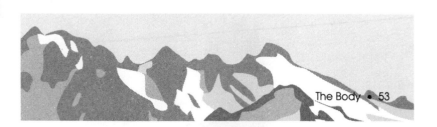

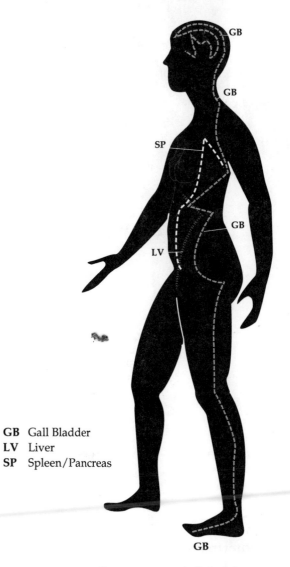

GB Gall Bladder
LV Liver
SP Spleen/Pancreas

ILLUSTRATION 4: SIDE MERIDIANS

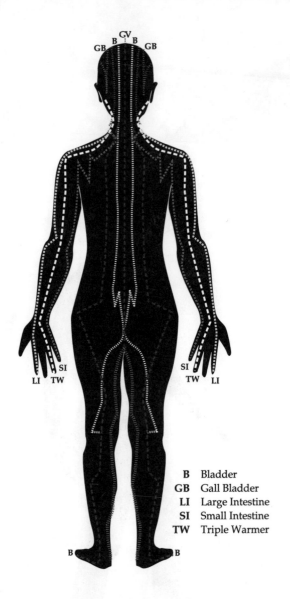

B	Bladder
GB	Gall Bladder
LI	Large Intestine
SI	Small Intestine
TW	Triple Warmer

ILLUSTRATION 5: BACK MERIDIANS

The Back

In Chinese medicine, the back is said to represent the past. The back takes the brunt from external, physical or psychological blows and it is defended, or armored accordingly. Through time,

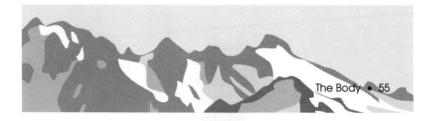

patterns of armoring are incorporated into the back's musculature, which is complex and multi-layered. This armoring can
eventually affect spinal alignment and/or the postural set of the
pelvic and shoulder girdles.

The back is defined energetically by the long sweep of the

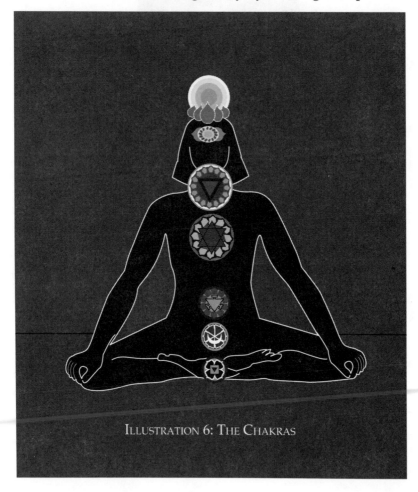

ILLUSTRATION 6: THE CHAKRAS

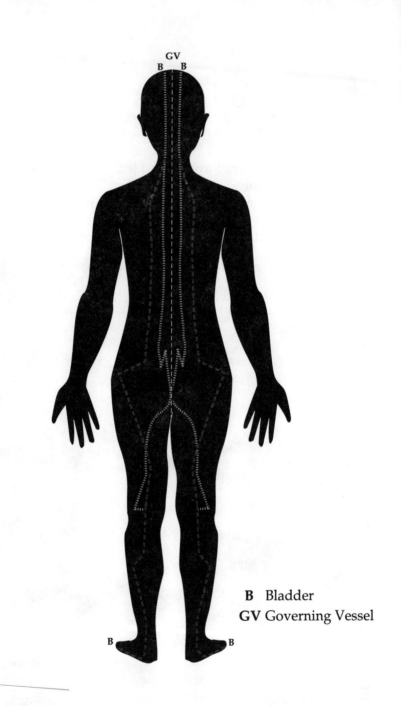

B Bladder
GV Governing Vessel

ILLUSTRATION 7: BLADDER MERIDIAN

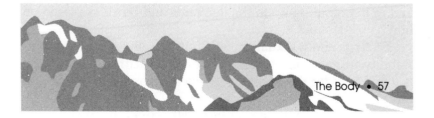

bladder meridian. (See Illustration 7.) This meridian originates at the inside corner of the eye, goes over the top of the head, and flows down the length of the back, in four pathways (including the two bilateral flows). It proceeds down through the legs and feet, ending in the little toe. There are some eighty acupoints (windows into the energy streams) of the bladder meridian along the back. It is thus not surprising that the back is such a fertile field for the storage of old hurts and subsequent patterns of imbalance.

One example of the storage of trauma in the back comes from a student:

> I realized that my back has been requesting a great deal of attention. I can feel a great tension all through my back from the mid-part of my neck all the way down to the lowermost regions... and the tension is spreading all the way around to the mid-part of my ribs. I realized with some tearfulness and anger how I was terribly assaulted about five years ago and never have worked that totally through. I was struck across the face, went down upon my knees and was struck with several blows to my back and lower neck....I notice how irritated I become when someone rubs my back....My back is almost telling me that it's time to come out, it's time that I become part of my front side and not treat my back as if it weren't there.

This student, fortunately, is now releasing the traumatic experience from his back through a combination of bodywork and psychological processing.

In addition to bearing its burden from the past, the back also undergoes the normal pressures of living. According to Alexander Lowen, the upper back carries feelings and pressures such as "demands of authority, duty, guilt and burdens both physical and psychological." The lower back sustains "an upward force through the legs supporting the individual in his erect posture and in his standing up to the demands and burdens placed on him."

Feelings about sexuality, self-control, self-support and self-stability are emotional forces that can travel up through the back. Is it any wonder that so many people have tension and pain in this area?

The bladder meridian, with its 80 acupoints on the back, provides access to these accumulated tensions. Acupoints within the region of distress may be worked directly to release pain and stress. But since the meridian is an extended energy flow— starting in the head and extending below the back to the feet— acupoints outside the specific area of stress can also release energy. Releasing the bladder meridian will automatically facilitate the release of stored psychic material, bringing both psychological resolution and the release of physical tension.

Interrelationships Between the Back And Various Organs

In addition to its direct relationship with the musculature of the back, the bladder meridian is related to other organic functions. Thirteen (26 bilaterally) "associated" points along, and just outside, the spinus processes relate to all the major body organs. There is a special point for each of the following: lungs, heart, pericardium, liver, gall bladder, spleen and pancreas, stomach, kidney, large and small intestines, the diaphragm and the triple warmer (signifying the three major energy centers of the body).

When the kidney point on the back is stimulated the kidney itself will be affected, in addition to the musculature of the back. Similarly, each of the associated points of the back can also affect corresponding organic functions and health. Through examining these points we may sense distress in the related organ and we may also help to relieve that distress. Our understanding of the bladder meridian provides us with an explanation of how back disorders are often translated into organic distress.

Energetic, muscular and postural release of the back is an essential part of freeing the consciousness since so much material is collected there over time and so many body functions are affected.

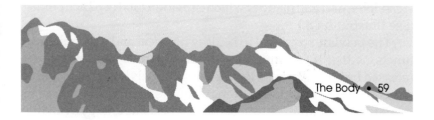

The Torso

According to Dr. Fritz Smith, the torso of the body (including the back) is "where we live." It is here that we hold the record of our lives. And, obviously, it is here that most organic functions are centered. The torso most completely reflects the core of the person.

The torso can be divided into several parts or "segments" that reflect different functional and psychological processes. In the following section, the principle "as in front, so behind" must be kept in mind. Thus, any disturbance in the front of the torso can be expected to cause stress in the back, often in an area directly behind the point of distress.

The Pelvis

The pelvis is a bowl-like, or "girdle" structure in the lower torso. It provides a structural foundation for the entire body. It also provides the critical connection between the torso and the legs and feet, through which "grounding" is achieved. The coccygeal and sacral vertebrae provide a channel for the nerves that supply the sexual energy that vitalizes the entire bodymind. Kenneth Dychtwald (1977) states that "its healthy and flexible functioning must be considered a necessity for a vital, free-flowing bodymind."

Pelvic Meridians

The pelvis is like the furnace in the basement of a large dwelling; it can warm the whole "home," bringing enthusiasm, creativity, pleasure and strength to the residents—but only if it is adequately fueled and maintained. Energetically, the pelvis is served by the first two chakras as well as by seven meridians—the large and small intestines, kidney, stomach, spleen/pancreas, liver, and gall bladder which provide a total of 62 acupoints. (See Illustration 8.)

The pelvis is so critical to healthy physical and psychological functions that it is sometimes the first part of the body to be released by bodyworkers. By releasing the pelvis the client is able to access the grounding, strength and stability she needs to establish a foundation for subsequent work. The energy available here provides confidence in one's sense of physical survival (first chakra). In Aikido training, this region represents the "base" of power, which must be securely connected with the ground.

The kidneys lie at the top of the pelvis in back. Their meridian flows from the feet up through the legs and all the way up through the front of the torso. In Oriental medicine, the kidney energy is believed to provide highly concentrated physical strength and energy. The kidney meridian is often strengthened first in acupuncture or acupressure, since it provides a strong energetic reservoir.

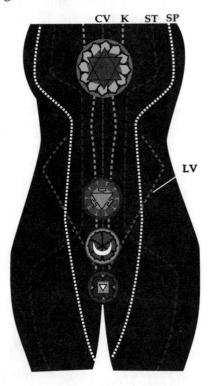

SP Spleen/Pancreas
K   Kidney
CV Conceptional Vessel
LV Liver
ST Stomach

ILLUSTRATION 8: PELVIC MERIDIANS

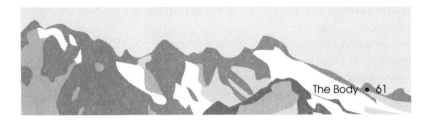

Elimination and Reproductive Processes

Two broadly important physiological functions originate in the pelvis: elimination and reproduction. These are highly susceptible to psychosomatic reaction. These functions roughly correspond to the first two chakras. The function of waste elimination from the physical body is accomplished predominantly through the large intestines, the kidneys and bladder. The large intestines and bladder organs are contained within the pelvic bowl or cavity. Their meridians also travel through the pelvis. Elimination of waste and toxic material from the physical body is critical to function and even survival; the body that cannot rid itself of waste soon becomes toxic and dies. The elimination of psychic waste—old stagnant ideas, bottled up feelings and the like—is also critical to healthy psychological function.

Freud associated the second stage of development—the anal stage, beginning at the age of two—with defecation. He theorized that the child who experiences disturbance in toilet training can become arrested in this stage, which brings about "anal-retentive" characteristics in the adult. These include the wish to hang on to one's own possessions, obstinacy, and cruelty to others. How toilet training has been handled helps to determine the individual's attitude toward punctuality, authority, neatness, doing one's duty every day and finally, holding on to things.

Similar characteristics are associated with the disturbed development of the root chakra (located at the base of the spine), which is seen as the seat of physical survival. Theoretically, the person whose life is threatened will kill to assure his own survival. The instinct for physical survival is expressed through forceful and raw aggression. These aggressive instincts are conditioned out of the child in its social development, but they can lodge as muscular armor, with attendant stored memories, in the pelvis.

Reproduction, with its great variety of physical and psycho-emotional complexities for people growing up in this culture, is associated with both chakras within the pelvis, although principally with the second. From the first stirrings of childhood sexuality, which Freud identified with oral gratification in infancy, through the turbulent period of puberty, extending into the adult reproductive years, a person may accumulate countless pleasurable and traumatic experiences of sexuality. The fixation on sex in this culture is an expression of the struggle to process and integrate these experiences. Much of this struggle is recorded in the pelvis. These experiences may include: sex play in childhood, the puberty development of sexual characteristics and activities (including masturbation, growing breasts, voice changes, etc.), first homosexual and heterosexual encounters, intercourse experiences linked with violation or rejection, childbirth, and extra-marital affairs.

The sexual experience produces both agony and ecstasy in most developing bodies, and all of this occurs within the pelvis. Many people simply cut off all feelings in the pelvis, in an attempt to gain control of the overwhelmingly confusing content of their sexuality. One student expressed it this way:

> *My pelvis actually feels excluded, like it's the black sheep of the body, the part that doesn't really fit. And the drive of my pelvis for affirmation and appreciation has been intense through the years, especially wanting men to be sexually attracted to me...but not really wanting sexual contact with them...but wanting them to want me....My pelvis really doesn't know much about its relationship with the rest of my body.*

Reich found people so cut off from their pelvises and their sexuality in his time that he built his entire theory of healthy function around the experience of orgasm—which involved the opening up or release of the pelvis. Specifically he claimed that the free body would experience streams of energy as a whole-body orgasm. He believed that this orgasmic experience was the key to a full and healthy life.

Many volumes have been written about sexuality in our time. Popular music, the consumer's market, and the entertainment

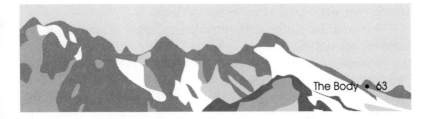

world—all owe much of their success to our preoccupation with sex. Yet this indulgence with sex does not produce pelvic health. Few bodies seem naturally free in the pelvis, able to express spontaneous, free-flowing movement, easy loving orgasm, and stable self-confident power from the body's base. It takes a great deal more than talk, sex games and entertainments, techniques and mechanical devices to assure the health and freedom which are the pelvis' natural heritage.

The Abdominal Region

The abdominal cavity, or belly, is the middle of the torso, bounded below by the pelvis and above by the diaphragm. It holds within it the major digestive organs (stomach, spleen, pancreas, liver, gall bladder and small intestines) as well as the internal branches of corresponding meridians. The area is therefore extremely vulnerable to outside influences, both through the digestive process and through physical impact. It is important to note that the digestive system is protected from the outside environment only by muscular walls. The abdominal region combines the abdominal and diaphragm segments in the Reichian (and Bioenergetics) systems.

Energy of the Abdominal Region

Energetically this area is served by the organ meridians already named above, along with the kidney meridian, which also runs through it. Thus, a total of six meridians and 42 acupoints (combining bilateral meridians) directly affect it. The third, or solar plexus, chakra is also located in the center of the region. (See Illustration 8.)

The abdominal region is functionally associated with digestive processes and, therefore, with the full range of physical nourishment. Energy blocks here can cause digestive dysfunction which will, of course, affect other systems.

This area also has broad psychological associations including most emotional expression. In some yogic traditions, it is called the "emotional brain," associated with personal power and the psychic sense of clairsentience.

Dychtwald called the belly the "feeling center of the bodymind," and points out that many emotions appear to originate in this region and then spread out through other areas of our bodies. He states, "When something is happening in our lives that gives birth to feelings, many of these emotions seem to "grow" out of our guts and will then spread outward through the rest of our bodymind."

The emotions of anger and fear, with all of their variations (jealousy, envy, anxiety, and the like) are especially strong in this area. Although they are recognized as primal emotions, anger and fear are stifled in our culture. A child learns very early how to "stuff" these emotions down into the belly rather than scream or tremble them up through the chest and the throat, and thus out into expression.

When the natural wave of emotion is not experienced and expressed, it becomes stored in the belly and congests that area with stagnant energetic debris. This debris may first be experienced as stress; later it can become fixed in place as armor. Over time the stress, or armor, can produce disease, both on emotional and physical levels, manifest as neurosis and chronic weakness or sickness.

Stored experiences within the abdomen were reported by a client:

> As I was being worked on, a series of experiences and memories unfolded. From the lower left intestinal area came memories of my last and very difficult pregnancy and anger at my husband then. Then anger, even rage about typing my husband's book and my father's presentation for a conference, anger at not being able to do it as they wanted, feelings of failing my father and being used without love returned.

When such old issues are cleared out of the energy system and the musculature of the abdomen, a person can regain the ability to know "gut level" feelings and be able to express them down through the pelvis and legs and up through the chest and

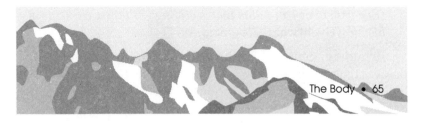

throat. A sense of personal power and ego strength ensues (founded from the free flow of energy through the third chakra), and the ability to assert oneself appropriately develops. One will know how to distinguish his own ego boundaries from those of another person. The person who is obstructed in this area will often get his own and another's feelings all mixed up. He tends to introject the other's emotions and to carry them within his own body. Therapists who are not trained in separating themselves from their clients, for example, often develop digestive problems or distended, fat-layered bellies as protection against taking on their clients' emotions.

Freedom in the abdominal region gives access to the natural gusto for life that is expressed through the "belly laugh" of Zorba the Greek. Food and feelings can be taken in and digested, and the person is able to allow these forms of nourishment to feed the bodymind.

The Chest

For our purposes here the chest is identified as that cavity of the torso framed by the shoulders at the top, taking in the rib cage, and culminating at the diaphragm on the bottom. It includes the upper back, the lungs and heart area as well as the heart chakra. Reichian work describes this section as the "thoracic segment."

The chest reflects a tremendous amount of psychosomatic process. According to Dychtwald, it is:

> ...primarily a feeling focuser, amplifier, and translator. Not only does it process the emotions that flow upward from the belly through the diaphragm but it also gives passion and inter-personal relatedness to these feelings. Because the chest is responsible for the harmonious integration of these varied bodymind aspects, it tends to shape itself in ways that reflect the

style with which an individual is dealing with these elements of his life. (Dychtwald, *Bodymind*, 1977)

Breathing, centered in the chest, is the first extra-uterine process that allows the newborn to make the transition between life in the womb and life in the outer world. It is also one of the last life processes experienced prior to death. The chest, therefore, expresses the full history of life, which may be reflected in layers of armoring.

Chest Meridians and Chakra

The depth and complexity of the chest is also displayed in the six meridians which traverse it—namely, the kidney, stomach, spleen/pancreas, heart, lung and pericardium. Each of these meridians gives further definition to the range of psychological experience possible through the chest, as does the heart chakra which lies directly in its middle. (See Illustration 9.)

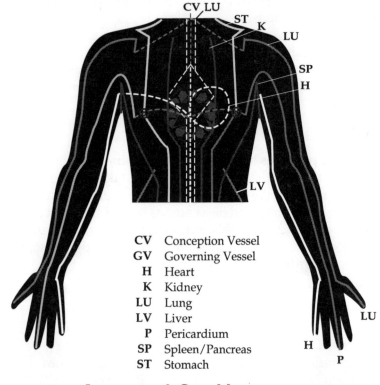

CV	Conception Vessel
GV	Governing Vessel
H	Heart
K	Kidney
LU	Lung
LV	Liver
P	Pericardium
SP	Spleen/Pancreas
ST	Stomach

ILLUSTRATION 9: CHEST MERIDIANS

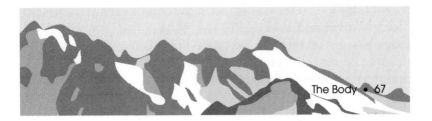

Breathing and the Lung Meridian

Although psychologists and therapists of various kinds have had many theories about the relationship between breathing and anxiety, Fritz Perls has made perhaps one of the clearest statements about it. "Anxiety is the experience of breathing difficulty during any blocked excitement. It is the experience of trying to get more air into the lungs immobilized by muscular constriction of the thoracic cage" (Dychtwald, *Bodymind*, 1977).

The powerful effect of breath release has been demonstrated in the last decade by "rebirthing" and the various offshoots of that process. These practices have revealed that a natural, full breath cycle is usually blocked at birth, or shortly thereafter, and is not regained until a process of conscious breathing reconnects it. It has been found that prolonged, systematic breathing will flush out stored psychic material and eventually reestablish the full breath cycle which will bring a person into a fuller sense of his own connection with Self and Spirit.

Lung Meridian

The lung meridian travels from the solar plexus, up through the midline of the chest, across the chest to a point at the upper lateral edge of the shoulder; and then it travels down the arm and ends in the thumb. The lung meridian is associated with the emotion of grief, holding on to old losses and/or grieving them unduly. In fact, working on the pathway of the meridian along the chest will often expose losses and sorrows of the past which have not been adequately grieved. For example, a colleague of mine was working this meridian in the body of a child who had been diagnosed as autistic, and who had not spoken or cried for seven years. At the Lung 1 point, located on the pectoralis muscle at the top of the edge of the breast (a particularly strong region of sorrow storage), tears welled up in the child's eyes and she said, "Mama" over and over again. Her mother had committed suicide just over seven years before! After this initial release of the original sorrow, the child gradually began to cry more, speak, and eventually began to laugh and play.

The Heart Meridian

The heart region of the chest includes the heart organ itself, its meridian, and the heart chakra. The heart meridian, which originates in the heart area, travels across the chest and down the inside of the arm into the hand, is known as the "Supreme Controller" in the Chinese system, describing its role as supervisor of the emotions. "The heart is the base of Life and home of the spirit. All consciousness and every thought belongs to the heart and the body is subjected to the heart like a country to its king" (Leung, 1971). The area is focused by a single point in the center of the sternum, Conception Vessel 17, which is called "spirit." In the Chinese system, as in other perspectives, the heart embodies the essence or individual spirit of the person.

The heart meridian is assisted in its task of supreme rulership by the pericardium meridian known as "the walled fortress of the heart." The energy of the pericardium encircles the heart and resides in the membrane which surrounds the heart. The meridian pathway also travels across the chest and down through the center of the arm into the palm of the hand, ending in the middle finger. The functions of this meridian are to execute the orders of the heart and to protect it, as well as to supervise blood circulation and kindle sexuality. Disease and trauma to the heart are said to be principally borne by the pericardium. That is, the protective wall of the heart sustains the external "blows" that would otherwise penetrate the heart directly. If the pericardium becomes too weakened and can no longer protect the heart, traumas may strike into the very essence of the person.

When this area is reasonably free, with an unobstructed flow of energy within the meridians and the chakra, a person experiences enthusiasm, inspiration, compassion, love and joy in living that come from Self-acceptance and contentment. Students report feelings of "gentle warmth and love," "bliss," "opening of compassion," and "transformation" when they are either giving or receiving work on the heart or pericardium meridians.

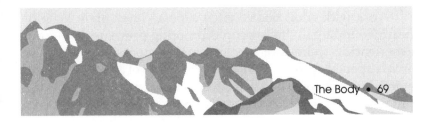

The Heart Chakra

As the heart beats continuously, renewing and sustaining the
physical body, so too does real love sustain and refresh us
spontaneously without outside stimulus. It is everflowing.
(Chitrabhanu, *The Psychology of Enlightenment*, 1979)

The fourth or heart chakra is associated with compassion, empathy and a feeling of oneness with all life. It offers a direct connection with the divine. Through it one can experience self-confidence, as distinguished from ego confidence. In yogic practice the opening and development of the heart chakra is a necessary step in one's evolution toward enlightenment. Great love for oneself, fellowmen/women and the divine must complement great understanding, else the seeker will become cold and un-feeling toward the human condition.

The heart region of the infant is usually open and free. The child experiences natural self-love, spontaneous affection and she reaches toward other people. But the heart is sensitive and easily wounded. Physical rejection, gestures of indifference and words of disapproval hurt the early tender heart. If such hurts persist, the child will gradually begin to pull back from heartfelt response and eventually take on self-protective, armoring patterns in the body.

Throughout my private practice and teaching I have yet to meet a person who was not wounded in the heart. The essential Self, expressed from the core, is loving and sensitive and natu-rally feels itself one with others, wishing to please them. It seeks approval, both to validate its own worthiness and to bring happiness to others. All too often, disapproval is used as a teaching tool in raising children. Continuous disapproval can wound the heart.

Work with adult bodies often exposes layer upon layer of heart wounding. In these people armoring prevents them from experiencing feelings of joy, love and compassion, unless the area is opened up again. "Opening the heart" of a client is greatly aided by a practitioner whose own heart is open, since the process requires the transformative power of free flowing heart energy, connected with divine love. In fact, heart wounding can go so deep, thrusting into the very essence, and into primal experiences of acceptance or rejection, that divine help often seems necessary. The bodyworker may wish to turn to spiritual resources in such a case. Profound healing work with the heart has been accomplished through prayer in the charismatic Christian movement (MacNutt, 1974); in the Inner Healing techniques of Ruth Carter Stapleton and others (Stapleton, 1977; Sanford, 1966); with Brugh Joy's heart-chakra-centered energy work (Joy, 1979); and in Jerald Jampolsky's Attitudinal Healing. All of these approaches call upon the power of the divine to intervene for deep, permanent healing. These techniques frequently effect miraculous resolutions and transformations that seemingly cannot be reached through ordinary psychotherapy. As Jampolsky (1980) expressed it, "I came to see that healing and love are inseparable."

The natural love which issues from and through the opened adult heart is not dependent on receiving affection from others. As Brugh Joy puts it, "the magnificence of the heart perspective of awareness is the direct connection to the divine aspects."

The Mid-Chest Chakra

Brugh Joy located a chakra which lies midway between the heart and throat chakras. In working with this energy center, I have found that it often reflects sorrows and losses in life. As long as the upper chest is stifled with these old sorrows, the free flow of emotional expression cannot rise up spontaneously from the lower torso into full articulation in the throat.

The free and whole person needs to be released from old sorrows that continue to restrict the bodymind, forming rigid armored patterns. In letting go of losses from the past, one can bring consciousness fully into the present and enjoy the fullness

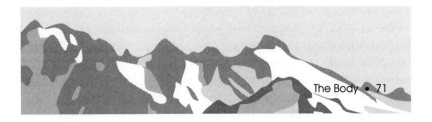

of life that is available now. Further, releasing old sorrows can give access to the full range of breathing, which rejuvenates the body's energy.

Neck and Throat

The neck and throat form a pathway, or bridge, between the body and the head. Through this channel the organic and emotional processes of the torso are relayed to the head. The nerve impulses that originate in the body are transmitted through the nerves in the neck up into the brain. Complex nerve and muscle trunks are bound together in this small area, which constitutes an extensive communication link in the bodymind.

The energy of the neck and throat are of high intensity. All six yang meridians of the body pass through the neck and throat; all of them cross at a single point (GV 14), between the seventh cervical and first thoracic vertebrae, where the neck joins the torso. In addition to the yang meridians, five yin meridians (lung, spleen, heart, kidney and liver) also send external branches up through the throat. In sum, eleven of the twelve organ meridians travel through this small area. Within this region, there are some twelve acupoints. Eight of them are called "windows of the sky," suggesting their capacity to open consciousness into higher realms. Further, the fifth, or throat chakra, is located at midpoint in the throat.

When there is congestion of energy in this area it can result in a variety of symptoms—tension in the neck, and a number of physical complaints such as sore throat, laryngitis, etc. Congestion may also manifest as psychological obstructions, such as the inability to express oneself creatively, or to speak up for oneself, to tell one's own truth, or to speak in public.

When acupoints of the neck and throat are congested, the

yang meridians, central channels (Governing and Conception Vessels), and the throat chakra are all correspondingly limited. The result is that energy and communication from the body does not pass easily into the brain. Thus, neck and throat congestion directly affect mental processes. Clearer thinking can often be facilitated by releasing energy through neck points.

Emotional impulses that originate deep in the body can culminate in conscious expression through the throat. For example, anger or fear, associated with the pelvis and solar plexus, can travel up through the chest and be released in vocal expression. The repressed person who is finally able to say "I am angry" has achieved a breakthrough in reclaiming his own power and ultimately himself. The fearful child makes a major step in handling fear when he can say "I am afraid." Completion or resolution of emotional tension often involves the throat region.

The Fifth Chakra

Creative expression, which begins in the second chakra, comes to fruition in the fifth, or throat, chakra. It is here that a person can express his or her own truth, generate creative ideas and finally gain the power of having a "voice," a unique identity. Personal and healing power can be projected through the "voice" by those adepts who have purified and mastered the instrument of their own creativity through the throat chakra. Swami Radha says, "When the voice is the magnet that attracts others, and a chord resounds in the heart of the listener, this is a sign that the aspirant is in contact with the Devi of Speech, with Sarasvati." Telepathy and the "extra-sense," clairaudience, also develops in the throat chakra.

There is an interesting reflection of the developmental stage of the personality in the voice. A child's voice is usually fairly high, melodious and innocent sounding. In puberty, the voice drops into a deeper tone. After a period of adjustment it usually settles, in adulthood, into a tone and style that it will keep for life unless it is trained in some special way. Some people retain an adolescent or even childish voice despite a wide range of expression which the actual voice instrument commands.

I have observed several times that when a person with a childish or adolescent voice gains insights, healings, and

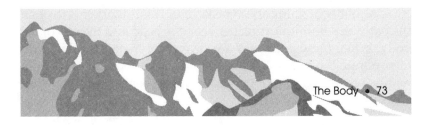

strengthening that allow him to "grow up," the voice becomes more mature sounding, as though matching the newfound maturity of its owner.

The Head

In a culture such as ours, which places a high priority on intellectual mastery, the head, holding the brain, is generally considered to be the person's master control center. The brain, with its trillions of cells and millions of possible synaptic junctures, is the "bio-computer" which ultimately controls most organic, rational and even emotional processes.

All higher mental processes are centered in the head. In addition, the senses—hearing, seeing, tasting, smelling—and the "extra-sense," of clairvoyance—associated with the brow chakra—are also focused here.

The head also embodies high energetic intensity. Six yang meridians, in addition to the Governing and Conception Vessels, cross over the head, which is punctuated by some 112 acupoints. The yin meridians of the liver and heart send internal branches through the head. The sixth (brow) chakra is located at mid-forehead and the seventh (crown) chakra penetrates the apex of the skull.

The free flow of energy in the head obviously facilitates a person's evolution toward a state of enlightenment. However, many people in our culture suffer from congestion or stagnation of energy in the head. We speak of a person who "lives in the head," meaning one who responds to life largely through mental processes that are not adequately connected with the emotions and bodily sensations that contribute to the unity of consciousness. A student reported, "Sometimes I feel that my head is cut off from my neck, and the neck sends messages to my head, and then I give myself headaches."

One of the first important tasks of the bodyworker is to open the paths of communication between the head and the rest of the body. When these pathways are clear the person's thinking can incorporate the valuable information signals coming to it from bodily sensation, emotions and psychic perceptions that full consciousness recognizes.

The Face Is a Window

The face is perhaps the single most expressive part of the body, since it shows our response to life through our eyes, nose, mouth, and the many tiny voluntary muscles of expression. It expresses our "mask" or persona. In youth, facial response is transparent, directly expressing the emotions of the child. Later in life a person may learn to control facial responses, usually as a defense against being "read," or known. The "stone face" of the criminal or judge is a good example of the armored face. Control of facial response, or a habitual expression, such as a grimace or smile, can result in fixed muscle tension and eventually, highly inhibited overall facial response. A student described his face as follows: "My face, in general, tries to put up a good front, but I've stored a fair amount of unpleasant feelings in the tense armoring around the eyes and cheeks. My smile is often defensive and insincere." The child who suppressed crying may become the man who cannot cry. Or the child who develops a perpetual pout may forget how to smile. Habituated expressions can be changed through bodywork or intentional training, such as acting classes. Psychic material and emotions that have been stored in facial muscles can be released and emerge into consciousness.

Jack Rosenberg, who works with Gestalt therapy techniques and facial release, has found that when facial musculature is released the person must be prepared to heal emotional material as well. An example of this phenomenon comes from a facial massage class he conducted at Esalen institute:

> One of the subjects receiving the massage began to cry and started into a very frightening (for him) reaction that centered about the feeling of being suffocated. As we worked with this terrifying emotion by Gestalt means, it became evident that he had regressed to a very early age—approximately six or seven— when general anesthesia had been forced on him for a broken

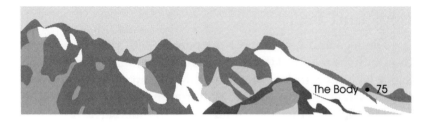

nose. All the fear and terror that had been there during those early years were again being expressed in the "here and now"—completely, and in a very real way. (Dychtwald, 1977)

A person who has released controlled facial patterns and who is committed to self-freedom can express a wide range of emotions in the face. A spontaneous response to life, in thought as well as action, may show again on the face as it did in childhood.

The eyes, sometimes called "the windows of the soul," are recognized by bodyworkers and psychologists as indicators of vitality, personal freedom and spirit. A person with little feeling of self-worth or identity, or who is heavily burdened with personal problems, will have dull or "dead" eyes that show no luster. Conversely, the person whose individual spirit is thriving will show vitality, "light" and depth in the eyes. The heart meridian, seat of individual spirit, sends internal branches directly into the eyes.

The Sixth and Seventh Chakras

The sixth and seventh chakras are traditionally associated with "higher consciousness," those abilities of direct knowing and of being attuned with the Universal order which have been sought by spiritual adepts through the centuries. The development of the brow chakra is associated with the ability to see through time and space, and to have a broader perception of life than one can perceive only through concrete data. The crown chakra gives a person direct access to Universal information and divine energy. According to Joy, only the crown and the heart chakras are directly connected with divine energy. Cranial work by a sensitive bodyworker can be beneficial in accessing the resources of these chakras.

Legs and Feet

The legs and feet connect the person with the ground and thus with the reality of the earthly plane. The torso rests upon the legs which carry it about in the world to accomplish its purpose. Six meridians flow up and down through the legs and into the feet, and all together they hold 124 acupoints. (Thirty-two of these points are known as "command points" because they exert powerful element-balancing influences on the whole bodymind.)

When a person is not grounded in the world, that is, unable to cope with, work with, and function in the environment and/or society, there is usually a corresponding weakness in the legs and/or feet. The weakness may or may not be manifest in acute conditions, such as disease or deformity. However, this weakness can be detected by the bodyworker as instability while standing or walking, or by the underdevelopment of the legs, the lack of feeling or sensation, etc. Alexander Lowen, originator of Bioenergetics, explained the grounding function as it affected the whole person:

> *Bioenergetically speaking, grounding serves the same function for the organism's energy system that it does for a high-tension electrical circuit. In the human personality the build-up of charge could be dangerous if the person were not grounded. The more a person can feel his contact with the ground, the more charge he will tolerate and the more feeling he can handle.... Finally, there is the anxiety of standing on one's own feet which connotes standing alone. As adults we all stand alone; that is the reality of our existence. But most people, I have found, are reluctant to accept this reality.* (Dychtwald, 1977)

When the life force does not course through the leg meridians the person experiences a sense of "spaciness," a lack of connection with earthly purpose, and a loss of confidence about his "stance" in life. A student related how she experienced her legs and feet:

> *I did not want to do this "present life" and the experience of paying attention to the legs confirmed a feeling I have had for most of my life of not really wanting to be here—one foot in the door and one foot out of the door, unable to move one way or the*

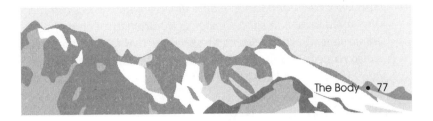

other through my arms and legs. The one fear I have is getting stuck like this in a sort of catatonia, a limbo that is neither alive or dead.

Stimulating energy through the legs brings a spacey person more into his or her body. Such a person is less likely to "fly off into the space of other times, other worlds," or to remain preoccupied with past traumatic experiences. As grounding is established, the person feels, and is, physically stronger and gains the stability to move forward into life.

There is usually less armor built up in the extremities than in the torso, and neck. This is perhaps due to the more continuous exercise and stimulation that the legs receive in the natural course of life. Even so, profound traumas can be stored here. For example, some Rolfers associate rigid fascia, on the inside and outside of the thighs, with mother and father experiences, respectively. When I received a second Rolfing series, I re-experienced my own birth as the Rolfer was working on my inner thighs. The most fascinating part of this experience was that as I felt myself being born, I also identified with my mother's childbirth pain, and I felt guilty about it, especially since I became aware of my actual resistance to getting born. I did not really want to come into this life. For many years the lack of life in my legs reflected this resistance.

Knee pain, swelling and weakness are common leg problems. The knees are often associated with fear, and with the need to bend to life's challenges.

In ancient Chinese medicine, the knees were felt to be related to the kidneys. The kidneys, in turn, were related to both the water element and the sexual organs. Water in this system relates to fear and correlates with the above. Our sexuality is related to our deepest vitality: forcing a man to his knees has always been experienced as humiliating. Going down on one's knees before a king or old person or sacred image is traditionally a sign of submission. We may reasonably speculate that locking the knees is also related. "I will not bend to your will." "I will not beg you." (Kurtz and Prestera, The Body Speaks, 1976)

Feet and Grounding

The feet provide our most concrete connection with the earth. When they are stable and aligned with the legs, we can take in energy and strength from the planet beneath us. The point Kidney 1, "Bubbling Spring," lies in the middle of the sole of the foot. Its name implies an energy connection with earth that can nourish us. In fact, it is one of the strongest emergency revival points in the whole human system.

When the feet are held in some position that obstructs firm contact with earth and legs, there is a corresponding psychological weakness in standing firm in life. I have observed several mystics whose feet do not make a stable contact with the ground. This lack of grounding can impede the ability to move forward with concrete purpose in ordinary life. One person described it as follows:

> My feet aren't comfortable. They try hard, feel inadequate and aren't fully joined with the rest of me. I feel like the inner edge is trying to hold on and figure out what to do, how to do it, while the outer edges are hardly on the ground, seem "flaky" in comparison. It is as though the outer edges have never matured into their full position and the inner edges are rather overcompensating (the kind of energy that was never young and takes things very seriously). There is no-boundary-ness, an energetic non-presence in the way the outer edges of my feet feel—they're flapping in the breeze, homeless.

When the feet fail to make good contact with the earth, instability is reflected throughout the rest of the body. In this respect, the feet give meaning and nourishment to the whole person. Dr. Fritz Smith once said that if the feet are not "open," allowing energy to course through them, work in the remainder of the body may not hold.

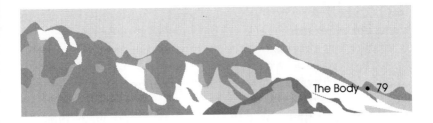

Arms and Hands

Just as our legs and feet connect us to the ground, so our arms and hands connect us to other people and to our actions in the world. They can extend out from us in almost any direction, as versatile "handlers" of people and materials. Dychtwald states:

> *The arms and hands provide the channels through which a great many functional emotions are expressed: they are able to transmit and generate such actions as hitting, stroking, striking, grasping, holding, taking, giving, reaching out, manipulating, feeling, self-protecting, and self-extending....They communicate the emotions, actions and functions of the bodymind to other people. (1977)*

Six meridians—including the lung, large intestine, heart, small intestine, pericardium and triple warmer—run up and down the arms and into the hands, with 61 acupoints on each side (totaling 122 points between the two arms). Thus part of the process and energy from each of these meridians (including their psychological associations) are worked out along the pathways in the arms and hands. Breathing, grief, elimination, assimilation (both physical and psychic) are all related issues of the arm meridians. Particularly important are the energy pathways from the heart (essence) and its protector (pericardium), since they help bring out into expression what comes from the individual spirit.

Weakness, imbalance or injury to the arms and hands may be associated with problems of connecting and doing. A Jungian analyst told me the story of how he came to psychiatry. He had been a surgeon. One day during surgery as he reached for the scalpel, his hand became paralyzed in mid-air. Nor would it move from the reaching position for several days. "That was the day I knew I was in the wrong work," reported this astute physician. After some weeks of therapy and a confirmed decision to change his profession, the paralysis disappeared and the strength of his hand was restored.

Reaching toward mother in infancy is one of our most natural acts, which progresses into reaching for other people in later life. If mother is not there, or if she rejects our touch, we may learn very early how to hold back within ourselves, not to reach out for others, and to avoid asking for what we truly want.

It is a natural desire to hold and to be held, to touch one another, to know each other kinesthetically. "Touching is a vital and exhilarating source of energy for me," one student reported. "I love to work with my hands, whether I'm digging in the earth, shaping clay or stroking a back." Many clients and students with whom I have worked are starved for that human touch which affirms them, makes them feel their bodies and allows them to share contact with each other.

The hands can be miraculous healing instruments. I have become convinced, through my work, that touching, holding, hugging and squeezing are kinesthetic anchors. We know, for example, that when babies are deprived of this touching, they can develop severe impairments or even manifest a "failure to thrive" syndrome. They can learn to do without and, finally, reject the very factor they need so desperately.

Finally, it is important to mention the shoulders as a bridge between arms and torso. The shoulders mediate between the emotional powers of the torso and the expressive powers of the arms and hands. In fact, the shoulders are associated with responsibility in general. We say, "he will shoulder the burden." Tensions and blocking here show that a person is carrying more responsibility than he is capable of handling. Eventually armor patterns can accumulate that will lock him into the attitude that life is a burden.

Historical Imprints Are Where You Find Them

After the basic survey of types of experiences that are commonly found in corresponding parts of the body, it is important to note that experiences can be stored in any part of the body; they

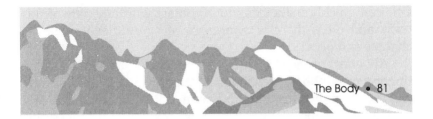

may show up in unexpected ways in seemingly unrelated areas. For example, I am reminded of the extraordinary recall of an experience that a woman reported about the violent death of her father. This memory occurred while her head was being worked on by the therapist. As her scalp and cranial bones were massaged her face contorted in agony. She reported:

I am looking at and feeling the violent crash. I see my father's body across the railroad tracks. I feel the shock and horror in my mother's body and consciousness as she witnessed his death.

This was a felt experience which resonated throughout the woman's body and consciousness, even though it was accessed through her head.

I believe it is even possible for experiences to be stored within the chakras or in the energy field around the body (aura). In any case, it is up to the therapist to maintain an open awareness, to take seriously whatever experience the client reports, and to be willing to *follow* that experience completely with the client as it unravels any place in the body.

The Free Body

The free body is related to, but not synonymous with, a healthy or fit body. Health in the body is generally defined by how its systems function at reasonable levels and the lack of serious symptoms. A "fit" body is muscularly toned, flexible and strong. The free body has been released from most of its character armor and consciousness has been thereby liberated from the major traumatic imprints of personal history. Such a body is vital, sensitive and awake to itself. It is the antithesis of the numb, armored body. Awareness is awake within it—proprioceptively, kinesthetically and emotionally. It is free to respond in the moment to the present reality of internal and external stimuli.

One can quickly make conscious contact with any part of this body and often there is awareness of specific energy flows, chakras and organs.

Aliveness of the free body is experienced through buzzing, tingling or bubbling sensations. It may feel like a mild electric current is running through it. Sometimes it can be seen internally as having streams or pockets of light. A student described this phenomenon as she was receiving bodywork: "I see clearly a straight line of light develop in my body as you work on me. Then that whole side of the body lights up. It's like the slow lighting of a neon tube." I have seen this experience myself and heard it described many times within bodywork sessions or trainings. Yet a free body is a fairly uncommon phenomenon in ordinary life. In fact it is rarely known apart from physically-engaged spiritual practice (such as yoga) or through armor release with bodywork that processes the corresponding personal history. Such a body is a joy to inhabit. It can grow stronger with age, rather than weaker as is common, and more receptive to the expression of the soul.

Summary

The body is the complete material substance of the whole person. As it develops from conception through maturity, the body records a huge variety of life experiences; these experiences are imprinted in, and help to form, the body. The physical record of life history accumulates in layers of armoring, from the deepest structures to the surface. These layers roughly correspond to the layers of the personality, namely, the core, the metaprogram, the body of personality and the persona.

Although the body operates as a whole, with all parts affecting all other parts, certain common experiences can be found in the armoring of each part.

The energy systems—meridians and chakras—give access to all parts of the body. It has been my experience that the release of these systems into the natural free flow of energy automatically brings about the release of corresponding armor and life experiences. Progressive release of armoring will eventually lead one back into the vitality and the information available at the core and in the soul's Master Program. With access to the soul and its true purpose, a person becomes fully self-actualizing.

CHAPTER FOUR

THE EMOTIONS

If emotion is neither expressed in its appropriate action
nor even admitted to consciousness,
it will have its revenge
by setting up some form of mental or physical distress.

—Weatherhead, quoted in Hall,
THE SECRET TEACHINGS OF ALL AGES (1977)

Emotions as Energy Waves

In Chapter One emotions were defined as an aroused state of the organism, involving conscious, visceral and behavioral changes. This aroused state includes the aspect of emotion as an electrochemical action which travels in waves throughout the entire body.

Western psychology recognizes basic emotions such as anger, fear and sadness. There are also extensive listings of emotions that include variations or extensions of these primary ones. Some psychotherapists work extensively with emotions on the premise that they are a viable part of human awareness and enjoyment. Others barely address them, contending that they simply get in the way of conscious direction. But there is as yet no organized field theory of emotions that relates them wholistically with physiological processes and mental and spiritual conditions.

An Eastern Perspective

Two ancient Eastern descriptions of the human organism offer maps for understanding emotions wholistically. They are the Chinese medical model of the five elements and the Indian yogic map of the chakras. Both systems are described in terms of energy. The Chinese medical model, first recorded in the *Nei Ching* in 200 B.C., outlined a system of emotions which related them to the five elements and the energy meridians of the body. The system follows the "natural laws" of energetic relationships within the body, mind, emotions, and spirit. It is the most comprehensive and most readily verifiable model of emotion I have yet encountered, and it provides a way to view and work with emotions that is congruent with all other parts of the whole person.

Ancient Indian yogic literature also classified emotions according to their association with the chakra energy system. The two energy maps—elements with their meridians, and chakras—provide a broad context for understanding emotions. I believe that together they form a complete view of natural emotional response, related to bodily, mental, and spiritual processes. Further, they give direction for a unified theory of emotions which allows us to identify where natural emotional response may be blocked, or which emotions may be excessively expressed.

All of the emotions related to the five elements are natural feeling responses to events—they give a healthy and rich emotional life. But within actual personality structures, we find that some emotions are expressed frequently while others seem curiously absent. It is also common for emotional patterns to run in families. For example, one family may express sorrow freely but rarely, if ever, express anger. This model of emotions allows us to identify root emotional complexes in the personality, and thus work with them appropriately.

I have chosen to work with emotions through the lens of these energetic systems because they consistently provide meaning to wholistic processes that can evolve toward self-actualization. Western psychological understanding can be integrated nicely within them as well. Dr. Leon Hammer's book, *Dragon Rises, Red Bird Flies*, is recommended as clinically describing these associations.

The Five Elements Theory

The five elements theory of Chinese medicine (particularly applied in acupuncture and acupressure) describes the human organism wholistically. The world and humans are seen through a cosmological grid of five basic elements, conditions or energies—fire, earth, metal, water, and wood.

The five elements system is a means of organizing and grouping concepts into a workable whole. It does not exist solely on its own, but represents the relationships of essential energies to each other....It helps to explain some of the physiological interactions among all these energies...(and) more generally describes man's relationship to the seasons and his physical environment.
(Matsumoto and Birch, *Five Elements and Ten Stems*, 1983)

This is an empirical system, drawn from observation of the human system and the world environment since before 200 B.C. The medical applications of the system, which were derived from a larger and older cosmology, were developed and tested through centuries of clinical practice.

The Chinese character which is traditionally translated as "element" can also be understood as "phases," "movements," "crossroads," or "path." Each element or phase represents an energy, archetype, or complex condition which spans the human energy system, many additional associations with the body, as well as various environmental factors such as season, climate and color. These associations are shown in Table 1.

The emotional associations with the elements are basic and minimal in the Chinese classics. Two qualifications for the application of the model in contemporary practice must be kept in mind: 1) evidence for the validity of these emotions as they relate to the meridians and organs of the body has been documented through 2,000 years of Chinese medical practice; and 2) new evidence for the model's applicability to Western contemporary man is being collected and documented by practitioners who are working with the theories (Teeguarden, Worsley, Connolly, Hammer, Raheem, and many acupuncturists). My presentation here is based on evidence collected from all these sources, as well as my own direct clinical experience.

As the student learns the associations with each element (Table 2), and observes them in people, she will form a sensory grid (visual, auditory, olfactory, proprioceptive) in consciousness which can be of great help in reading and assessing a client's needs.

The Energy Systems and the Emotions

In the following sections emotions will be linked to the elements and their meridians. We will first explore the relationships between the clusters of emotions and the elements and meridians. Then we will explore how specific emotions are associated with specific chakras. Emotional states associated with elements, meridians and chakras overlap, of course, since the large energy vortices of the chakras feed into the energy streams of the meridians beneath them. The descriptions of emotional states are, in our discussion, separated out for clarity, but as the student becomes familiar with the body and its energy systems, emotional interactions between meridians and chakras will become obvious.

Working with emotions as they manifest through the energy systems consistently reveals certain principles and patterns.

PRINCIPLES OF EMOTIONAL/ENERGETIC REACTION

1. The energy systems, including meridians and chakras, provide the capacity for a full range of emotional expression. This broad complex of emotions provides a guide for fully experiencing life at a healthy emotional level.

2. When energy flows in the meridians and/or chakras are balanced, a characteristic "centered" or "appropriate" emotion

will be expressed. (Each of these centered emotions is described, as it relates to its particular element, in the following sections.)

3. When energy flow becomes imbalanced—toward excess or deficiency—an exaggerated emotion is expressed. Exaggerated emotions fall at both sides of the centered one, for example, hysteria/sadness, sympathy/self-absorption, grief/refusal to grieve, fear/bravado, anger/apathy.

4. Energy imbalances can cause emotional imbalances and emotional imbalance can cause energy imbalance.

5. Energetic/emotional imbalances can become habitual over time, and thus continue to reinforce imbalance.

6. Habituated energetic/emotional patterns can bring about a fixed emotional pattern within the personality wherein a particular set of emotions would be frequently expressed while others would rarely, if ever, be expressed.

The Five Elements Theory and the Emotions

The *Nei Ching* named five emotions associated with the five elements. These are: joy, sympathy, grief, fear and anger. These five emotions provide a simple grid which enables us to identify the primary emotional complexes that are organically and energetically rooted in the body. Each of the five can be further amplified into a cluster of related affects, which range from "balanced" to "imbalanced" emotional expressions. For example, joy is the balanced expression of fire, whereas sadness (lack of joy) and hysteria (too much joy) are imbalanced expressions of it. The five clusters taken together include the full range of all major and subtle emotions. Yet, any one emotion can be linked to one of the five elements, which enables us to identify and assist primary wholistic needs within the bodymind/emotions. (Teeguarden has worked extensively with the five elements model of emotions as it can be applied to Western bodies. She has identified the clusters of emotion associated with each element in detail in her book *The Joy of Feeling*.) Each of the primary emotions associated with the five elements, together with their related emotions, will be explored in the following sections.

The five elements—fire, earth, metal, water, and wood—express their energy through twelve organ meridians. Four meridians are associated with the fire element, while two meridians are associated with each of the additional four elements. The flow of energy between the elements forms an interlocking, continuous circuit. (See Illustration 10.) Thus, whatever affects one part of the system will eventually affect all the parts. When emotional response is free, and events are met appropriately, the elements are maintained in a healthy (and fluctuating) balance. If one element is frequently overused, or conversely repressed, imbalance within it (and eventually within its companion elements) will ensue. As the elements and their emotions are described in the following sections, this integrated wholeness must be kept in mind.

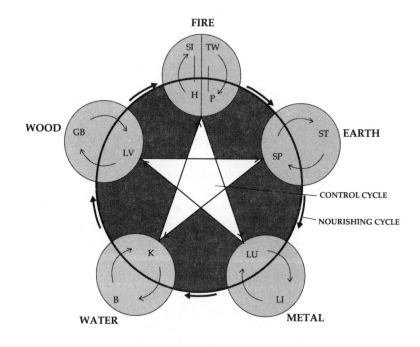

ILLUSTRATION 10: THE FIVE ELEMENTS

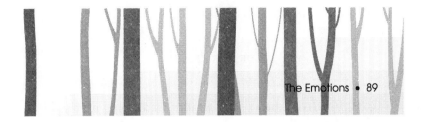

Each of the elements has many associations, in addition to the emotional ones, that show the body's energy condition. These include: smell, taste, flesh color, tone of voice, a sense organ and a part or system of the body. In addition to these body associations, environmental ones, including season, climate, planet and type of growth are useful in showing how the human system is affected by the macro-environment (see Tables 1 and 2). These indices are often helpful in reading the emotional state, as well.

THE ELEMENT	WOOD	FIRE	EARTH	METAL	WATER
Direction	East	South	Center	West	North
Season	Spring	Summer	long summer	Autumn	Winter
Climatic Conditon	Wind	Summer Heat	Dampness	Dryness	Cold
Process	Birth	Growth	Transformation	Harvest	Storage
Color	Green	Red	Yellow	White	Black
Taste	Sour	Bitter	Sweet	Pungent	Salty
Smell	Goatish	Burning	Fragrant	Rank	Rotten
Yin Organ	Liver	Heart	Spleen	Lungs	Kidneys
Yang Organ	Gall Bladder	Small Intestine	Stomach	Large Intestine	Bladder
Opening	Eyes	Tongue	Mouth	Nose	Ears
Tissue	Sinews	Blood Vessels	Flesh	Skin/Hair	Bones
Emotion	Anger	Happiness	Pensiveness	Sadness	Fear
Human Sound	Shout	Laughter	Song	Weeping	Groan

TABLE 1: CORRESPONDENCES OF THE FIVE ELEMENTS

TABLE 2:

THE FIVE ELEMENTS

Compiled from many sources and traditional materials

THE ELEMENT:	1 FIRE	2 EARTH

MERIDIANS:	Heart (H) (I)
	  Small Yin
	Small Intestlne (SI) (II)
	  Great Yang
	Pericardium (P) (V)
	  Absolute Yin
	Triple Warmer (TW) (VI)
	Small Yang
		Spleen/pancreas (Sp) (XII)
		  Great Yin
		
		Stomach (St) (XI)
		  Middle Yang

NUMBER OF POINTS:	H: 9, SI:l9, P: 9, Tw: 23	Sp: 21, St: 45
TIME:	H: 11 am-lpm, SI 1-3 pm P: 7-9 pm, Tw: 9-11pm	Sp: 9-11 am St: 7-9am
SEASON:	Summer	Indian summer, between seasons
CLIMATE:	Hot	Humid
COLOR:	Red	Yellow, orange
OFFICIAL OF:	Emperor (H), Sorter of pure from impure (SI), Heart Pro- tector (P), Heat Balancer (TW)	Digestion of life, food, protection, energy transportation
PART OF BODY:	Blood, vascular system	Muscles, flesh
SHOWS CONDITION OF:	Complexion	Lips
SENSE ORGAN & SENSE:	Tongue, speech	Mouth, taste
BODY FLUID:	Sweat	Saliva
SMELL:	Scorched	Fragrant
VOICE:	Laughing	Singing
SOUND:	F, Ha, Ho	A, Hu
LIFE ASPECT:	Spirit	Ideas, opinions

3 METAL	4 WATER	5 WOOD

Lung (Lu) (IX)
  Great Yin
	Kidney (K) (IV)
	  Small Yin
		Liver (Lv) (VIII)
		  Absolute Yin

Large Intestine (LI) (X)
  Middle Yang
	Bladder (B) (III)
	  Great Yang
		Gall Bladder (GB) (VII)
		  Small Yang

Lu: 11, LI:20	K: 27, B: 67	Lv: 14 GB: 44
Lu: 3-5 ams Lu: 5-7 am	K: 5-7 pm, B: 3-5 pm	Lv: 1-3 am GB 11-1 am
Autumn	Winter	Spring
Dry	Cold	Wind
White, black	Blue, black	Green
Receiving chi, eliminating waste	Water balance	Creation, Planning, Decision, Judgment
Skin, body hair	Bones, marrow	Tendons, ligaments
Body hair	Hair on head	Nails
Nose, smell	Ears, hearing	Eyes, vision
Mucus	Urine	Tears
Rotten	Putrid	Rancid
Weeping	Groaning	Shouting
0, Saaa	U, Chui, Fu	I, Shu (Hsu)
Animal Spirit	Faith, courage	Will

TABLE 2:

THE FIVE ELEMENTS

(Continued)

ELEMENT	1 FIRE	2 EARTH
SPIRITUAL MANIFESTATION:	Spirit	Intellignece
PROCESS:	Growth	Transformation
EMOTIONS:	Joy, hysteria, sadness	Empathy, worry, obsessions, self-absorption
PERSONALITY:	Active	Calm
TEMPERAMENT:	Emotions up and down	Obsessed
TASTE:	Bitter	Sweet
FOOD:		
• Excess counteracted by:	Salty	Sour
• Tonify with:	Pungent	Salty
• Sedate with:	Bitter	Sweet
• In disease, requires:	Sour	Salty
• Beneficial cereal:	Millet	Rye
• Beneficial meat:	Mutton	Beef
OVERUSE INJURES:	Use of eyes	Sitting
IN EXCITEMENT, CHANGES, CAUSES:	Lack of joy, compassion	Belching, Obstinacy
GOVERNS:	Divine spirit	Ideas, opinions
PLANET: • Associated with:	Mars Pioneer, innovator	Saturn Natural dignity and authority

3 METAL	4 WATER	5 WOOD
Aura	Aspiration	Soul
Harvest	Storage	Birth
Grief, letting go, holding on	Appropriate fear, paranoia, foolhardiness	Will to become, anger and lethargy
Simple	Likes movement	Hard working
Anguished	Fearful	Depressed
Pungent	Salty	Sour
Bitter	Sweet	Pungent
Sour	Bitter	Sweet
Pungent	Salty	Sour
Bitter	Pungent	Sweet
Rice	Beans	Wheat
Horse	Pork	Chicken
Lying down	Standing	Walking
Grief, sadness, cough, rejection	Trembling, release of tension	Control, decisions
Animal spirit	Will power, ambition	Spiritual faculties
Venus Sensuous enjoyment, wars & jurisdiction, Uranus	Mercury Basic intelligence, especially of dangers and retreat	Jupiter Magnanimity, gentleness

Element: Fire; Emotion: Joy

The element known as Fire is related to a broad range of qualities that characterize its natural state: warmth, quickening, transformation. It can be symbolized by the archetype of Spirit—that eternal flame from the Source which sparks the individual, bringing inspiration and meaning to life. In the physical body, fire is associated with the circulatory system, the tongue, a scorched smell and a bitter taste. Psychologically, it relates to spirit, intensity, intuition, joy and laughter. Fire stimulates the energies of increase, growth and space. Red is the color attributed to fire and summer is its season

Joy is the emotion associated with fire in the *Nei Ching*. When fire energy is balanced in the system one experiences a natural joy of being oneself and has a zest for living. When fire energy is too low, one experiences sadness, a lack of joy. When fire energy is too high, one may experience hypertension or hysteria. The full gamut of emotions associated with fire has been identified by Teeguarden in *The Joy of Feeling*. They cover the range from hyperexcitement, elation and hope at the strong or excessive pole, to sadness, discouragement and depression at the weak or deficient pole.

Fire energy is reflected in four meridians: heart, small intestine, pericardium and triple warmer. Together these meridians govern the balanced play of fire qualities within the body, mind, emotions and soul. Each one of these meridians supervises certain physical and psychological functions, as follows:

The heart meridian is called the "Emperor" in traditional Chinese literature, denoting its power over the circulatory system and its rightful place as supervisor of all the emotions. It is known as "the dwelling place of the spirit" (*Nei Ching*). The individual spirit is what manifests our unique expression of the divine flame. Inspiration and intuition, functions of the heart, can keep us attuned to the transcendent guidance available to us beyond the promptings of the personal ego. The person who lives from his own spirit or heart will have access to the joy of being true to himself (see table).

The heart meridian radiates out from the heart center in three directions, resembling a flower that opens across the chest. One path originates in the heart center, travels across the chest and down the inner arm into the hand; another travels from the heart up through the throat and to the eyes; the final path descends from the chest into the torso. These pathways describe the energetic means for feeling one's own spirit's truth and joy (in the heart center); for perceiving from one's own center (through the heart and eyes); and for expressing from the spirit (through the throat, arms, and hands).

Many spiritual teachers have emphasized "seeing and feeling with the heart." American Indians described the strength of a warrior as "having heart." Some cultures, including the ancient Egyptian, described the heart as the center of one's being.

An Egyptian mantra, taught by Nadia Eagles of the Egyptian-Huna lineage, exemplifies this belief: "My heart, at the perfect moment, unfolds the soul and plants the seed for the mountain of me to come forward."

In our hearts we carry our own individual spirits. Inspiration and intuition, associated with the heart and fire, help us to remember that spirit. And this spirit comes forth from each of us in a completely unique way. To come into individuation one must follow one's own heart, one's own fire, and one's own spirit—in short, to follow what brings joy to our hearts is to follow the self.

As Emperor, the heart should be in control, that is, supervising all emotional expression. The Emperor needs to allow the play of emotion and yet maintain final authority over that play. If emotions go beyond appropriate expression and begin to damage the balance of the whole system, then the heart, as Emperor, must assume control and, guided by the spirit of wisdom and intuition, once more command balance and bring the person into alignment with his own individual spirit. Such management, arising from the wisdom of the heart, would assure the truth-sensing support of the emotions, but prevent a person from being overcome by them.

According to the *Nei Ching:* "Because the Shen (Spirit) has such intimate connections with the emotions, any emotional stress will also affect the heart."

BALANCE IN FIRE

If the fire meridians and organs are sound, then there will be adequate blood circulation to feed the entire system with oxygen and nutrients (the basic fuels) to maintain healthy bodymind/ soul/emotions. Spirit will flame up, in inspiration. The contentment and joy that comes from expressing one's own heart will be easily accessible. There will be abundant laughter. And the Emperor will be strong, to guide a person through the appropriate evolution in this life.

IMBALANCED FIRE

Characteristically, a person whose fire is burning low experiences sadness. He has become alienated from his/her own heart and loses access to the deepest wisdom of individual spirit. There is insufficient joy and inspiration in that person's life.

Loss of fire can develop over a period of time when the heart has not been validated. Heart wounding starts very early in life, when the first threats to selfhood begin; parents may not validate the essence of the child; peers may tease and denigrate him. Eventually he will incorporate others' negative evaluations and so develop a negative self-concept.

On the other hand, excessive fire in the system can also cause imbalances in emotional responses. When there is too much fire a person may become hysterical, laugh excessively, and be overly subject to impulsive action. Continuous excessive fiery emotion and action from the heart can literally cause a person to "burn out," a condition well known in the helping professions.

FIRE ENERGY AND THE PERICARDIUM

An interesting aspect of the energy associated with fire is that the heart organ and meridian receive protection from the pericardium membrane and meridian (sometimes called "Heart Protector" or "Heart Constrictor"). This meridian surrounds the heart and sends a branch of energy down the inside of the arm close to the heart meridian. It has been traditionally described as the protective wall that catches potential wounding blows aimed at the heart.

Continuous emotional assault over time can exhaust the pericardium meridian until it loses its ability to protect the heart. Without the shield of the pericardium the heart may receive hurts directly into it. Here we have a model, in the energy system, for safe emotional development: the heart or individual spirit does indeed need protection, particularly in childhood, until there is sufficient ego development for self-managed protection.

The pericardium meridian is also called Circulation-Sex, which denotes its function as regulator of intimate relationships and sexuality. An internal branch of the meridian goes down along the midline from the heart center toward the pelvis and second chakra region. The fire of sexual impulse and response is thus directly fed by the energy of the heart and pericardium, and by the openness of the individual spirit. When fire is weak, and a person is cut off from the qualities of his spirit, intimate relationships cannot be adequately "warmed."

The Link Between Heart and Small Intestine

In addition to the protection it receives from the pericardium meridian, the heart is assisted by its mate, the small intestine meridian, which provides both assimilation and discernment functions. As the official who "sorts the pure from the impure," the small intestine meridian deepens the heart's wisdom and helps to refine its discernment, by directing a continual assimilation process that keeps what is useful and true within the system and discards what is not helpful.

The small intestine meridian runs up the outer arm from the little finger, across the scapula, up through the neck and ends in the face. An internal branch runs down the front of the body into the region of the small intestine organ, which is responsible for digesting and absorbing usable nutrients and sending undigestible materials on to the large intestine.

The Triple Warmer Meridian and Social Relationships

The last of the fire meridians, triple warmer, is related to regulation of body temperature, metabolism and "social relationships," that is, those connections with others beyond the one-to-one relationships of intimacy. As we warm in the "three burning spaces" of the triple warmer (chest, abdomen and pelvis) we are fully enlivened to relate with others at all levels of human experience. (These "burning spaces," of course, are directly associated with the first four chakras, which we will consider in the following section.)

The triple warmer meridian begins in the ring finger, ascends the back of the arm, over the elbow and up through the shoulder joint to the top of the shoulder blade, and further ascends the neck, travels up through the occiput and along the side of the head behind the ear and ends above the eyebrow in the forehead. It also sends a branch of energy over the top of the shoulder and down into the torso in the front of the body to create the three warming spaces of respiration, digestion, and elimination.

FIRE AND DEVELOPMENTAL FACTORS

The young child often lives close to his own spirit. He expresses himself through full-bodied spontaneity. His joy bubbles out in laughter. He is warm and quickly responsive to both pain and pleasure. As his spirit is acknowledged and respected by caring parents he will gain confidence in the validity of his own feelings and his own worth. He will feel: "I am welcome here as a worthwhile and valuable person."

The fortunate adult, whose heartfelt feelings and joy in living have been validated through family and society, can be true to his own individual spirit, speak the truth of that spirit, and enjoy life fully, with warmth and laughter.

Often, however, as life unfolds, the child can sustain wounds to the heart, ranging from simple rejections to severe hurts that will gradually cause the build-up of defensive emotional behavior and armoring of the heart center and the chest. Armoring and habitual withholding patterns can eventually result in the person being cut off from his own heartfelt responses to life. "Anguish and fear are injurious to the heart," says the Nei Ching. The person who can no longer sense his own spirit, nor feel joy and love, will become sad.

Continual sadness leads to insufficient energy within the fire element (which can eventually lead to heart organ disorders), lack of ability to give or receive love, and a general sense of purposelessness. Chronic subliminal depression can result from prolonged depletion of fire energy. In later life, such a depression can turn to bitterness or cynicism, as well as heart or heart-related diseases.

Element: Earth; Emotion: Nourishment

The element Earth holds within it those qualities we instinctively attribute to the ground beneath us—stability, protection, food, center and balance. Traditional associations with the element which also help to delineate its nature are: the season of Indian summer, the color yellow, a sweet taste and smell, the mouth, muscles, a singing voice and the energy of transformation. The stomach meridian, which feeds earth, is known as "the sea of nourishment."

Sympathy is the emotion associated with earth in the *Nei Ching*. In psychological terms, empathy is a more accurate word since it connotes understanding and warmth for the problems of others, rather than pity and identification with them, which we usually associate with sympathy. As I discuss it here, earth is additionally associated with a variety of emotions related to nourishment and connectedness. The cluster of emotions within the earth element ranges from the balanced state of sympathy or empathy, through the imbalances of self-absorption or narcissism, to over-identification with others.

The energy of earth is expressed in the body through the organs and meridians of the stomach, and spleen/pancreas. The location of the organs in the solar plexus—the middle of the body—reflect the quality of balance and stability in the earth element.

The stomach meridian is known as the "official of nourishment," while the spleen (pancreas) is called the "official of distribution" (of nourishment). The stomach, assisted by spleen and pancreas, receives and helps to process nutrients. These meridians also have bearing on our intake, output and transformation of other forms of nourishment; warmth, contact and support from others.

The path of the stomach meridian moves down the front of the body, from head to toe. The spleen (pancreas) meridian pathway begins at the end of the big toe and travels up the front of the body, framing the abdomen and chest and ending at the side.

The stomach meridian's full downward sweep constitutes an energetic course for complete grounding, bringing energy from the head and face, all the way down into the feet. It also follows the direction of digestion, from the mouth through the abdomen. This meridian is literally a diagram on the body for "earthing" or "grounding," that is, for connecting the person with the earth in a way that stabilizes and nourishes. Grounding gives reality to physical support from the earth. When the pathway is open there is vitality in the digestive process, as well as a stable energetic sense of connection with the earth in the legs and feet.

Earth can be associated with the archetype of the mother in all her forms—the divine Mother; the personal mother; the earth as mother, that primal bed of our existence; Mother Nature, the abundance of life support on earth; the mothering energy within others; and finally, the mother within us who will ultimately direct the process of getting our deepest needs met toward self-fulfillment.

BALANCED EARTH

When earth is healthy, one experiences connectedness to others and holds them in warm positive regard. There is an ability to empathize, or know how to "walk in the other person's shoes." One wishes to be caring, and to nourish the needs of others within reasonable limits. There is also a healthy respect for one's own needs, and the know-how to gain nourishment for them. Ego boundaries are appropriately established within the concept of relating to others. In a broader sense, there is sympathy for the human condition in general. In optimum earth development a person has a stable sense of grounding or security with oneself, with others, and with the planet.

IMBALANCED EARTH

If the earth element is imbalanced, a person may express emotions at the extreme ends of the continuum—i.e., either she is completely self-centered, cut off from the needs and sufferings of others, or she is obsessively identified with others to the exclusion of self-needs. Further, the person will probably swing from one of these imbalances to the other in the progression of an earth disorder.

Self-absorption, or narcissism, occurs when a person feels emotionally undernourished. This condition almost inevitably develops from a situation of incomplete, absent or abusive mothering. There is a continual drive to fill an inner vacuum of inadequate mother love, through searching for mother substitutes and self-indulgences of every kind. Such a person may withdraw into herself to continuously "nurse" and enlarge internal feelings or needs. The feeling of disconnection from others may be guarded and accentuated by the accumulation of excess fat on the body, which functions as a way to insulate or keep a distance between herself and other people.

At the other extreme of earth imbalance we have the nurturer-helper who identifies deeply with others and may become obsessive about their needs, to the exclusion of her own. Ego boundaries can dissolve when one identifies so deeply with another person that feelings merge. When this happens it becomes difficult to separate consciousness of self from that of another person. Many helper-healers become over-burdened with the problems and conditions of their clients, exhausting their resources, and are then subject to an earth imbalance.

EARTH AND DEVELOPMENTAL FACTORS

The infant's first life connection is with the personal mother and the life-sustaining nourishment of breast milk. (Stomach point 17 lies directly on the nipple of the breast.) Shortly after birth the fortunate infant is put to its mother's breast where its own sucking instinct draws nourishment through life-giving contact with mother. This contact will become a prototype for later connection with others.

The process of breast feeding gives nourishment, satisfies the sucking instinct and provides physical contact with mother's body as a continuous bonding process. Resting into mother's body, directly over the stomach meridian, the infant can again feel and hear mother's heartbeat, her vibration, her warmth—all factors which reinforce a sense of physical security. In this way a visceral experience of nourishment and safety is imprinted into the core of the body. Freud theorized that when this first oral gratification is provided, a basic sense of security is established. When it is not provided—as in cases when infants are removed from adequate mother or surrogate-mother contact—the resulting insecurity can create arrested development in the oral state, with oral fixations. The visceral memory of mother nourishment and safety can be restimulated later in life through sensitive and loving touch from another. It is one of the factors that makes knowledgeable bodywork deeply effective.

When caring nourishment—physical, emotional and energetic—are established in infancy through a full opening of the earth element, there is automatic trust of the mother and the environment. The child learns that there is safe support on earth. He experiences the prototype process of that support: crying out, receiving the breast and finally, drawing in the nourishment through sucking.

Throughout life the development of connectedness to others is promoted through the earth element. In infancy, we are attached and wholly dependent upon mother and develop trust through her. Later dependence and awareness can be extended towards others—father, siblings, greater family, peers, teachers and others. Gradually the child gains a base stability and trust from these dependencies, while practicing her ability to draw in nourishment. From dependency she will move toward independence and gain the ability to ask for what she needs from others. From being nurtured she will eventually develop the ability to give other people nurturing. Out of a base of nurtured strength, she will have the capacity and wish to support others.

In optimum earth development, the adult will learn how to become her own mother. She will find ways to nourish herself in all aspects—body, mind, emotions and spirit—in such elements as nourishing food; touch for the body; nurturing emotional and mental impressions from art and music; and spiritual food through spiritual practice and commitment. Complete dependence on others for basic survival needs (as in childhood) is transcended and one can become astutely competent at getting what one needs. Obviously, dependence on others is a natural part of the human experience, since we are a social species, yet in adulthood our basic guidance system needs to originate within the Self, and not from the personal mother or mother surrogate.

Few people in our culture have enjoyed complete mothering—abundant nourishment, bonding and a sense of safety. For this reason one of the important functions of therapy is to teach the client how to cultivate the mother within herself, who can take over the nurturing functions.

The phenomenon of dependence, or transference, of a client to the therapist is one of the principal issues in most therapy. As support and guidance are received by a client (sometimes for the first time) she may seem to develop an appetite for nourishment that is virtually insatiable. The more the helper gives, the more the client (or friend, lover, etc.) wants. This appetite can continue through many years of therapy if the therapist does not help the client move through the deprived baby stage to adulthood. Freud theorized that there is a wish within all of us to return to the womb and the comfort of infancy and stay there, receiving endlessly. If therapy, or a relationship, is to truly assist growth, it must evolve into a peer relationship, in which the person eventually learns to draw nourishment and guidance from within and develop an independent ego.

The responsible therapist will deal with the earth element directly as soon as it is appropriate within the therapeutic process. This may include searching out the root of the earth imbalance (which will quite likely be in early childhood), correcting or healing it, and then working to strengthen the client so that she can draw from her own earth energy within and from the planetary earth energy.

Element: Metal; Emotion: Grief

The element metal is characterized in the macro-environment by structure in the earth, form, "heaven" and the Autumn season. Within the human system it is associated with a white or silver color, the skin and hair, the sense of smell, a pungent taste, a rotten smell, a weeping voice and a balancing energy. The classics claim that "heaven" chi, or energy, is brought into the body through the breath.

The emotion of grief is associated with metal. Grief is distinguished from sadness (lack of joy in fire), and it is understood as the healthy response to separation from what has been dear to us. The cluster of emotions within metal ranges from rigid withholding of emotion and possessiveness to excessive grieving over what has already been lost.

Metal is expressed through the organs and meridians of the lungs and large intestine. The lung meridian originates as an internal flow of energy in the stomach region then flows up through the lung area and across the upper chest, then down the arm, ending in the thumb. The large intestine meridian arises in the index finger, travels back up the arm, across the top of the shoulder, up through the neck and into the face.

The lungs and large intestines, and their meridians, provide the function of elimination, with the lungs eliminating carbon dioxide through the breath cycle, and the large intestines eliminating unused wastes from ingested nutrients. The skin, also associated with metal, provides yet another whole body system of elimination.

An emotional elimination process—letting go—is also associated with the metal element. We take in the "heavenly spirit," or "space" of the cosmos (Tao) with the inhalation. We let go of old, worn-out feelings and burdens of the past through exhalation of the breath and elimination through the skin and large intestines.

Metal can be associated with the archetype of the father in the spiritual sense of father as the one who gives structure, guidance and "heavenly" attunement. The lung meridian has sometimes been called the "priest within the temple," whereas the large intestine meridian is the "janitor within the temple."

WHEN METAL IS BALANCED

The balanced emotional condition of metal is one of acceptance, surrender and harmony with the environment. This feeling provides the necessary awareness of when to "let go" when something has been taken away. The breathing process provides a model for the free flow of feeling in a balanced system. As we breath in, we take the material elements (oxygen, etc.) and cosmic energy or life force of the environment into our lungs and lung meridian, thus connecting us in that moment with the very atmosphere which sustains us.

As air and life force (chi) are circulated within us, the life processes are fueled, and consciousness is integrated with that moment's cosmic reality. And finally, with exhalation, we let these effects pass through, neither holding on to any moment's nourishment or experience, nor grieving unduly over their loss after they are gone.

The natural grieving process of separating and saying goodbye to what we have lost is part of the balancing of metal. In fact, within the metal element we have a most useful model for that process as widely taught by Kübler-Ross. We have learned that the traditional way of responding to loss with stoicism (withholding of feelings, rigid non-expression) results in emotional and physical problems later on. Feelings of sorrow stay locked in the body. But when we allow a period of grieving, freely expressed through crying, we can honor the meaning of our loss and wash the residue of sorrow out of the body. As we accept and express the grieving, there is finally a period of letting go. The body and feelings are finally clear and free; then we can return to an open state, to accept the incoming flow of new life and new connections.

The cluster of emotions associated with metal is beautifully congruent with its seasonal quality. As autumn yields its fruit, so the person who is healthy and whole in the metal element will yield to the flow of events, offering up the fruits of his labors, flexible and yielding in the process and ultimately surrendering to the divine order.

IMBALANCES IN THE METAL ELEMENT

At the opposite poles of balanced metal lie the complexes of withholding (of feelings) and rigid holding on (in the body) or, at the other extreme, excessive grieving over loss. These two conditions arise from either an "excess" of energy or matter (unusable toxins) within the metal element, or a deficiency or poor quality of energy or matter therein. Examples of the holding process are: constipation in large intestines, the tendency to hold emotion in the chest (impaired breathing) and holding fast to old beliefs and ideas. Excessive grieving is the opposite quality of sorrowing over what has been lost, which eventually can degenerate into a state of "crying over spilt milk." This condition weakens the metal element.

A person who has a respiratory ailment such as pneumonia, asthma, or even a cold, will have congested lungs, filled with excess mucus, with stagnated energy in the lung meridian. Similarly, a large intestine obstruction will result in extra waste material in the organ and an excess of energy in the corresponding meridian. A person will tend to be contracted in the body, breathing shallowly and/or will be unable to eliminate naturally and easily. When either one or both of these physiological conditions exists, consciousness will be correspondingly affected. The toxic quality of old thoughts and feelings is held in the body. The person can become locked into rigid belief systems and outmoded structures, defending those beliefs and refusing to acknowledge the freshness of changing realities.

When the full metal cycle of taking in and letting go is denied, a person may develop a metal imbalance that can manifest in chronic lung or large intestine symptoms. Grief can accumulate within the body, manifesting as chest armoring or lung organ or meridian congestion, if losses are not grieved appropriately at the time. Conversely, prolonged sorrowing can weaken the metal element. Either of these ways of dealing with loss can become habituated, which further reinforces an imbalance. The person with a weeping voice, who sighs and tends to cry frequently (or conversely, not at all) often exhibits a chronic imbalance in metal.

Element: Water; Emotion: Fear

The water element is characterized by fluidity, cold, damp, the color blue and the winter season. It is expressed in the body through the organs and meridians of the bladder and kidneys. The bladder meridian, as we have previously discussed, makes a broad sweep down the full length of the back, and is associated with storing memories of past experiences. (See Illustration 6.) Its mate, the kidney meridian, runs from the bottom of the foot, up the inside of the legs, and into the chest. The kidney meridian controls the physical strength of the body, including its sexual energy, and as such is closely connected with the first two chakras, which provide the impetus and guidance for survival and sexuality.

Fear is the emotion associated with water in the classics. The term includes a wide spectrum of related emotions, such as awe, wonder, respect and timidity. Courage and steadfastness are expressed as a balanced water state, whereas terror, fear and paranoia are expressed as one imbalanced polar extreme, with foolhardiness, or excess bravado at the opposite pole.

Water can be associated with the archetype of the Warrior who is strong in body and mind and who has learned many ways of facing and steadfastly struggling with obstacles. The Warrior is aware of dangerous realities. He does not foolishly deny what can be harmful but rather than shrinking from threats he takes them as challenges to refine his strength and develop his skills of alertness and will.

BALANCE IN WATER

Teeguarden has described the balanced condition of water as "awareness of relativity," by which she means appropriate fear responses to life-threatening events. In other words, one can accept the reality of danger and act cautiously and appropriately, without collapsing in the face of it. Fear is a necessary and life-preserving response since it stimulates action for survival.

When the water element is strong and stable one has a basic strength and endurance. There is awe, even reverence for the natural order of things, and a healthy respect for danger. Out of such strength we find the courage and faith to meet life's events with vigor. Natural stresses and problems are handled with confidence, as creative challenges and resolutions are effected.

The water element gives strength to our resolutions. We have the steadfastness required to keep trying, to follow through and carry things to completion. Without this feeling of strength and mental focus a person cannot achieve life goals and purposes.

WATER AND WINTER

Water is associated with the winter season and here the Chinese provide sage guidance for health and well-being. As demonstrated in nature, winter is a time for contraction, for going inward. It is a time to rejuvenate, to strengthen at the roots. After a long season of growth, it is time to retreat into the quiet darkness, to gather resources and fortify ourselves for the coming year. In this we have a model for tending the water energy; after a creatively productive period, a period of effort to expand outward in a day or week or year—we must take time to restore vital energy within the water element and the core of the self. Thus we build physical strength, emotional courage and faith to prepare ourselves for another spring.

WATER IMBALANCES

A person whose water energy is low automatically experiences frequent fear. Ordinary stresses and problems seem threatening and one may lack confidence in resolving them. Threats and stresses of contemporary life are subtle but continuous, with massive toxicity in the environment and constant information and events that stimulate anxiety. A person with strong water energy can navigate through these challenges; the fear response will provoke energy to solve them. But to the person with low water energy (and this is a fairly common condition, in my experience), most problems and challenges can seem insurmountable. As one fear is resolved, through analysis or action, another will pop up to take its place. In fact, it is not possible to dispel the underlying tone of fear in the person whose water energy is low. Over time, unresolved fears tend to emotionally paralyze such a person, resulting in a water depression marked by chronic anxiety.

Through the Chinese system of medicine we learn that a person is not capable of intellectually resolving a fear until his kidney energy is strengthened and stabilized. I have discovered in my practice that countless therapeutic hours can be saved by recognizing this fact. I have made it a practice to strengthen the water energy substantially before tackling the resolution of chronic or deep-seated fears.

When the kidney energy is fortified, the person who is fearful of every event and threat that life offers will automatically become more confident and hopeful and will gain the ability to view threats as obstacles to be creatively overcome.

A person with imbalanced kidney energy—at the "foolhardy" extreme—may take unnecessary risks, placing himself in situations that are dangerous either physically or emotionally. Over time excessive effort and risk will exhaust the kidney energy and throw the system into the opposite extreme, of weak water energy and a response of fear.

The bladder meridian is emotionally important in relation to past fears. Physically and energetically it is closely related to the kidney meridian, its mate. Throughout its long path along the back, it can collect past fears. These can influence a person's response to current situations. For example, a person who experienced abuse in childhood may continue to react from his fear of that time to events and relationships in the present even though they are no longer abusive. Fear can be introjected from the body of another, particularly the mother's. A client who was extremely aware in her body reported that she could locate her mother's fear in her own bladder meridian.

As the back and bladder meridians are released, these old fears will come to the surface. They can be examined in consciousness, resolved and healed. Then the person regains strength for the present that is no longer conditioned by past fears.

Element: Wood; Emotion: Anger

The element wood signifies growth in all its aspects. The sprouting proliferation of new life in springtime is symbolic of this creative, expansive energy. Associations with wood in the bodymind are: anger or assertiveness, the color green, the eyes and seeing, ligaments and fascia, a shouting voice, a sour taste and rancid smell, and the energy of birth or rebirth.

The gall bladder and liver meridians express wood energy. The gall bladder meridian frames the body from head to foot, principally along the side. The liver meridian ascends from the foot into the lower torso, culminating in the mid-torso area.

Wood could be represented by the archetype of the Divine Child who emerges through a process of rebirth. Just as husks from the withered branch contain seeds that will sprout new life, our human experience covers over, and holds within it, the seeds of new growth. Transformation from the personality into the soul, or the Divine Child, can come about as useless patterns and frozen imprints of the past are discarded, revealing the pure new growth potential underneath. Eventually, rebirth into the soul is possible.

Carl Rogers observed that a "lead growth shoot" within each person finds a growth path (even if a distorted one) through all obstacles. Just as the seed contains the blueprint, or pattern, for the full tree, so the soul carries the blueprint for self-actualization. Carl Jung called this growth potential the "root of consciousness."

> What is capable of transformation is just this root of consciousness which—inconspicuous and almost invisible (i.e., unconscious) though it is—provides consciousness with all its energy. (Jung, *Modern Man in Search of a Soul*, 1933)

It is fascinating to note that the Chinese associated the term "soul" with the liver meridian. The heart meridian, as we saw, is related to the "spirit." I have pondered these associations extensively. My own speculation is that the soul aspect aligned with the liver is that immortal, divine seed which is stable from life to life and which carries the evolutionary record, whereas "spirit" (heart) relates to the individual (Self) development of a given life. In the 5-element cycle of nourishment, liver nourishes heart, just as the soul essence must feed our individuality.

Wood is associated in the classics with anger. However, the word "assertion" can perhaps better serve, since it implies the thrusting force that pushes us toward growth and rebirth into the self. Assertion helps us to push through environmental restrictions toward the Divine Child potential. The cluster of emotions associated with wood range from apathy, through assertiveness, to rage.

BALANCED WOOD

The balanced state of wood brings purposeful direction, or what Teeguarden calls the "will to become." This condition is one of controlled growth, where a person is guided by his own vision and is able to take deliberate action towards creative goals. Self-assertion is a necessary part of this actualization process. Appropriate anger, in response to being hurt or thwarted in our growth, is also a natural and healthy expression of wood. When anger is allowed to be expressed in its natural flow, it blows over quickly and clears the air. Only when it is held down and accumulated in the body does it become destructive.

The creative drive to fulfill the self and its purpose is analogous to the thrusting energy of wood. Creative developments result from progressive stages of growth that fill out destiny. For example, focused intention, a quality so crucial for creative productivity and manifestation, and determination are aspects of wood energy. Blocked creativity produces anger and frustration which, when stored in the body, will eventually cause lethargy and aimlessness.

IMBALANCES IN WOOD

At opposite poles of the balanced state of wood are rage at one end, and apathy at the other. Within these extremes there is a variety of expression: aggressive feelings, irritation, frustration, blame, resentment, and guilt.

The expression of anger is discouraged in our culture, whether it is appropriate or not. Therefore, anger is often held within the body where it becomes distorted and leaks out in unconscious hostility. The prevalence of violence in the media is one expression of the pent-up unconscious anger we carry as a society.

A person who is imbalanced in wood may be irritable most of the time, with occasional outbursts of rage. His anger is old, seldom related to the here and now. Much of his energy is dissipated in these feelings (which attach to whatever stimuli are available) and thus drive is lost for purposeful creative action. As energy is depleted in useless anger over old issues, the wood element can become weakened, resulting in loss of hope and apathy.

When wood energy is weak a person will have difficulty manifesting his own life purpose and meaning. The depression which results from imbalanced wood energy can be one of deep despair, in which one cannot find one's way.

WOOD IN DEVELOPMENT

While connection and nourishment from mother are worked out in the earth element, I have often found a relationship with the personal father in the wood element. The positive personal father traditionally provides guidance, direction and discipline to the growing child. His clarity of vision, and his ability to create a structure for the realization of that vision, can demonstrate how to plan and execute worldly tasks. Eventually the outer discipline imposed by the father will become self-discipline. The fortunate child of such a father can call upon a fund of developed skills within himself and he will gradually learn how to direct his own development to go on toward self-fulfillment.

Fathers have been absent from the lives of many children in the last several decades, as a result of high divorce rates and increased single parenting. Without a strong father figure, a child may feel the frustration and anger of being inadequately guided. It can be difficult to develop skills of envisioning, planning, finding meaning and direction in adulthood without an early formative father model. Resentment over father deprivation supplants the purposeful hope that a good father can instill. When these qualities of fathering have been missed in development, it is extremely helpful to strengthen the wood element and teach skills to a person so that eventually he may develop the father within, who can guide the growth process.

About Love

Love is not associated with one particular element but is understood as a more global phenomenon that derives from all of them. As we experience and express the "fire" or passion of love, other emotions frequently fuel that fire. Certainly sympathy (earth) is aroused for the beloved; we are able to place her happiness above our own. Love helps us let go of old sorrow and surrender into the here and now (metal). Love may provoke fear (water) of losing the loved one but it will also stimulate our courage to pursue the relationship. Finally, we are stimulated toward renewed purpose, creativity, and meaning (wood) during the blossoming of love. As explained in the next section, love is related specifically to the heart chakra and its energy is known, through experience and literature, to be one of the most powerful cohesive and healing forces in life.

The Cycle of Elements and Emotions

As shown earlier, the five elements form a complete system of energetic/organic interaction. Balance within one element engenders or nourishes balance within the next element, or conversely, imbalance within one tends to progress to the next. (See Illustration 9.) Emotionally this cycle can be expressed as follows: Joy (fire) is natural as we follow the truth of our own individual spirit. Joy nourishes our ability to have sympathy, or empathy (earth) for ourselves and others. As we are nourished and grounded in earth, we have more capacity to flow with the natural order of life (metal). Acceptance of life as it is engenders the faith, courage and will to persist (water). Acting with courage builds our assertive power to move forward with growth (wood). And following our "lead growth shoot" brings joy (completing the full cycle back into fire).

Imbalances, of course, progress similarly through a negative cycle: Sadness (fire) weakens the capacity for sympathy (earth). Without empathy and nourishment we tend to get stuck in old emotions and events (metal) which diminish our capacity to act with strength (water). From a position of weakness and fear we grow apathetic (wood) and are unable to grow freely, which further saddens us (fire).

The Chakras and Emotions

The chakra wheels of energy describe much larger and more generalized areas of the body than do the meridian streams. Their energy vortices feed into several meridians at once, which they both influence and are influenced by. Paying attention to the chakra energy therefore gives a more global sense of a person's basic orientation to life in the present and as it has developed over time. Through a reading of chakra energy we can quickly locate the basic emotional character of a person. Rama, Ballentine and Ajaya have called the chakras the "centers of integration," which is an apt description of their major consolidating functions. By further reading the specific meridians that stream out from the central chakra system, we can delineate more exact origins and effects of emotional character (Illustration 6).

The Root Chakra

The root chakra is located at the base of the spine in the perineal floor. It is associated with the anus and the coccyx and is understood to form the base of the chakra system. Within this base three primal energy pathways arise and flow up the spine: the sushumna, a central flow; the *ida,* arising from the left, and *pingala,* arising from the right. These latter two flows crisscross at each chakra as they travel upward, until they meet in union at the sixth chakra. There is also a locked store of energy within the root chakra—the kundalini, or coiled serpent goddess as it is some-times depicted—which energy lies dormant until it is released

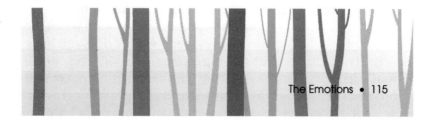

through unusual means.

The root chakra develops fully in the first seven years of life. It is influenced by anal issues. According to Freud, voluntary control of bowel movements is the first full act of self-control, and it establishes a base of selfhood, or sense of one's own power. Toilet training and the protection, or violation, of the anal area contribute to either a basic sense of security or a basic fear of annihilation.

I have found that the root chakra energy is often related to how well a person has connected with the protective strength and endurance of the father. If the child is grounded in the body by parents and an environment that make him feel safe and confident of his own body identity and strength, then he will have a solid energetic base and skills development for dealing with the rest of his life successfully. His "survival instincts" will be firmly rooted. According to Rama, Ballentine and Ajaya:

> When a person has his energy centered here (the root) he will be concerned about being hurt by others, not only psychologically but in a physical sense. The fear involved here is an intense, unreasonable fear of the magnitude that is associated with the role of the hunter and the hunted. It is a total and global sort of anxiety. (Yoga and Psychotherapy, 1976)

If the root chakra is developed (through early parental grounding and/or specific physical practice such as yoga or the martial arts), a person will feel confident of his ability to cope with physical life. Abundant energy can flow from the root into the legs and feet, reinforcing the sense of connection to the earth and life purpose. Such a person can feel proficient in survival skills and know how to "land on his feet."

The kidney and bladder meridians are fed by this chakra. As noted, they bring basic physical strength and courage when their energy is strong, or fear when it is not. Fear is also associated with the root chakra. Similar to the automatic fear caused by a weak kidney meridian, fear becomes the prominent emotion when the root chakra is not adequately developed, when it does not have the vitality, radiance and staying power that we find in the martial artist, for example. A person with a weak root chakra will understandably be fearful for his survival and physical well-being. Out of that fear he may disregard any life except his own and resort to ruthless violence to protect himself.

The Second Chakra

The second chakra is located over the genitals and bladder area, between the navel and the pubis. It is related to the genitals, sexuality and the creative impulse in general. While the root chakra controls the sense of self-survival, the second chakra dictates species survival, through procreation. Sensual pleasure is the focus of this chakra, together with the multiplicity of feelings that drive us toward sensuality. Raw sexual impulse is one of the primary seeds of creativity. The energetic strength in this chakra provides stamina to generate and sustain creative production. The kidney meridian, also the seat of sexuality, runs through it.

Second chakra energy is developed primarily from ages 7 to 14. The most primal genital issues—acceptance of sexual identity and feelings about one's specific genitals—originate during this time and within this chakra. The feelings generated here are intensely pleasurable and they can enliven the body completely when they are allowed to flow freely. The orgasmic potential can increase fire in the system (feeding the meridians of pericardium, heart and penetrating channel), and thus stimulate joy. The joy-pleasure of uninhibited sensuality can act as a powerful impetus toward growth.

Such a potential is not automatically available in normally conditioned bodies. Taboos about experiencing and accepting genitals, sensual exploration and natural sexual development generally lock this potential up in belief-bound and armored bodies. In fact, both natural and developed sexuality (as in some hidden forms of tantra yoga) are difficult to locate in our culture. Locking this energy away not only prohibits the renewing joy of sexuality but also diminishes our creative impulse in all areas.

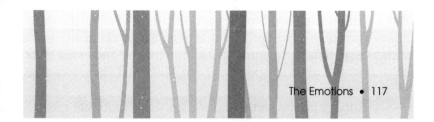

The Third Chakra

The third or solar plexus chakra, is located at the navel. It is traditionally associated with digestion, assimilation and personal power, and is regarded in the yogic tradition as the center of physical energy. This chakra feeds into, and draws from, the earth meridians (stomach and spleen/pancreas) and wood meridians (liver and gall bladder). It helps to consolidate both earth and wood energies, and thus subsumes their emotions of empathy and aggression.

According to Rama, Ballentine and Ajaya, this center is concerned with effective and assertive individual behavior which will permit one to provide for one's personal needs—clothing, shelter, and the securing and digestion of food.

Once again we are looking at the most primal nourishment needs. When they are met, a person will feel confident and competent and can develop an adequate personal ego. But if they are not met a person can feel inferior and develop an inferiority complex which can lead to either dominating or submissive behavior.

As with the element earth the manner in which a person connects with others is often guided by the third chakra. Exaggerated energy in this chakra can cause one to place his own needs and ego above everyone else's. Such a person can become narcissistic, overbearing and obsessed with personal power.

A neglected third chakra can result in a lack of personal power, the inability to assert oneself, inadequate ego development and the loss of ego boundaries.

The confluence of mother and father relationships form the basis for the development of ego and personal power. Both male and female discipline and support are required for the full flowering of the personal ego. I have found that mother and father relationships need to be worked through before the third chakra can fully develop. When a person can claim her own mothering and fathering qualities within the self and enlist their aid to develop a strong personal ego, the third chakra can be greatly strengthened.

The third chakra is sometimes called the "emotional mind." It is known to affect how a person identifies with others. If ego boundaries are weak, one can "absorb" the emotions of other people directly into the body through this chakra. In such a case, one may "take on" both emotional and physical problems of other people.

The Heart Chakra

The heart chakra marks a developmental transition from the lower three chakras into the upper four. It is located over the chest, between the breasts. It is fed by the heart and pericardium meridians and thus relates to joy and the expression of individual spirit. Beyond individual joy and fulfillment, it also opens the capacity for true self-love and true love of others. In fact, it is at this center that our evolution progresses from the basic self-survival impulses of the first three chakras into transpersonal aspirations given by the upper three chakras. Within this center the "lower" and "higher" capacities of the human being can be integrated. Further, right and left sides of the bodymind, representing the active, yang, masculine qualities and the receptive, yin, feminine qualities are also integrated in this center. The universal symbol of the cross finds its centerpoint in the heart. An energetic organization around this center potentially involves the whole person.

Higher forms of love, compassion and unconditional love originate in this center. These forms of caring for others go beyond possession or attachment. Compassion is traditionally associated with the Buddha, Christ and most great spiritual teachers. Somewhat beyond empathy, this love is only possible when one has a sense of inner fullness and no longer craves for much outside the self. As the heart chakra develops, one can begin to become integrated and whole within oneself, and have less need to merge with others in order to regain lost or projected parts of oneself.

Mothers often feel and give unconditional love, attention,

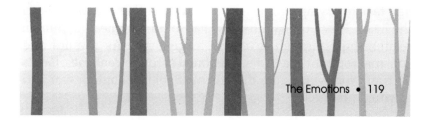

comfort and care to their babies without expecting anything in return. As a mother holds a baby to her breast, it is nestled directly over the heart chakra where it can soak in her love energy, which is critical for the infant's development. Infants who receive unconditional love have the most valuable foundation for healthy development. Conversely, those who do not receive it are undernourished in fire from the beginning, and their capacity to give and receive love in later life will be limited until they can fully experience unconditional love. The heart and pericardium meridians both send branches of energy down through the arms and into the hands. When we hug another person with an open heart we are literally "wrapping" them in loving, healing energy.

Divine Love and the Heart Chakra

Unconditional love is not often available through people. The heart development required for it generally occurs only after deep spiritual practice and commitment to the service of humankind. Fortunately, the healing and nourishment we need from such pure love is available from God. Divine love can be sought and received directly through the heart and crown chakras. The charismatic Christian healing tradition, and many other heart devotional and spiritual paths, are based on the reception of divine love, or Grace.

There are many examples in contemporary literature where people with physical and/or emotional heart conditions—which seemed medically or psychotherapeutically irreparable—received divine healing with a complete cessation of all symptoms.

Even when the physical body cannot be cured, emotional healing can occur through divine love. Jampolsky reports many children and adults with terminal cancer who have received this grace. Similarly, Kübler-Ross claims that the single most important task for dying people is to deal with unfinished business of the heart. Much of that business has to do with healing human relationships through love and forgiveness. As mystics and spiritual aspirants have demonstrated through centuries, God's love and forgiveness are directly available through prayer and spiritual practice.

The Throat Chakra

The fifth or throat chakra progresses transpersonal capacities of service to others that were opened in the heart. Whereas love is the principal expression of the heart, truth, derived from actual experience in the body and heart, can be delivered through the voice. The throat chakra has to do with creativity and receptivity. Emotion does not originate here, but feelings from the lower chakras can be brought to resolution and completion by expression through the voice. Here feelings are refined, tempered with love from the heart, and expressed with compassion as creative acts.

Healing abilities are associated with the developed throat chakra; it is here that loving energy from the heart can be focused with the word. In fact, the voice itself can become an instrument of healing through truth-telling in song, lecture or everyday speech.

When the throat chakra is open and receptive, the person experiences a feeling of surrender, calm acceptance of the greater order beyond the personal. While the ego, and its evolution or growth, is the principal focal point for the lower three chakras, the opening of the throat chakra may include transcendence of that ego into higher spiritual awareness. As the throat chakra is developed, a person realizes and welcomes the possibility of harmonizing the personal ego with the great infinite order. In Christian terms, the development of the throat chakra heralds the ability to say "Thy will (not mine) be done." It is easy to see, then, why the feelings associated with the developed throat chakra are tranquility, acceptance and assurance.

The Sixth and Seventh Chakras

The two upper chakras do not generate emotion. They govern mental and spiritual faculties and in the yogic tradition are said to be "beyond emotion." Their fields of consciousness include the capacity for being aware of emotion without being bodily involved with it, or electrochemically influenced by it. As viewed from the perspective of these chakras, emotion is seen as an integral part of human reality, but it does not "grip" or "sway" that higher consciousness.

Emotions and Body Armor

The electrochemical charge of emotion that is freely allowed and felt in the body brings heightened vitality and awareness. It will naturally flow to completion through expression. However, when discharge of emotion is blocked, by denial or inhibition of expression, its charge can be stored in body tissue where it will become a barrier to the free flow of energy and emotion later on. Such stored emotional charges are the building blocks of body armor, which, as we saw in Chapter Three, begins to form quite early in life.

Early emotional responses are simple: fear, anger and something akin to affection, or "drawing toward," can be observed in the newborn. These seem to be innate; they provide the infant's primal response to basic life supports and life experiences. In the vulnerable, undefended body, these emotions are ideally expressed instantaneously and freely, flowing through in a wave-like motion from beginning to completion in a short time, then released from the body. It is not widely understood, however, that frustrated primal responses (for example, an infant's screams of anger at not being fed) are often recorded in the body and can be retrieved from it some 20 or 30 years later through deep bodywork. When emotion is stopped in its course, as when the child is not allowed to cry, then residual effects are stored in body tissue, or "stuffed," as we refer to it in process psychology.

Conditioning will alter the free expression of emotions as the child grows. Socialization requires rage to be muted and fear responses to be curbed. As these stops or revisions of emotional expression are imposed by the outside world, the child learns to hold the energetic charge of emotion within the body rather than scream or cry it out. Over time these pockets of unexpressed emotion can become energetic charges locked in tissue. Such emotional incompletions are incorporated into the body as neuromuscular patterns of "armoring."

Emotional Health

Emotions are an integral part of human consciousness. They provide natural bodily feeling responses to life events. They help us to sense what's going on in the environment and indicate how our bodies can accommodate these realities in a healthy way. The variety and range of emotions in the free body is wide and they charge us with interest and vitality. The process of self-realization or individuation requires extensive awareness and development of emotional states. They give both sensitivity and energy to our human journey and help us find the next steps in growth.

Emotion is the chief source of all becoming-consciousness. There can be no transforming of darkness into light and of apathy into movement without emotion. (Jung, *Psychological Aspects of the Modern Archetype*, 1938)

Through the energy lens of the five elements, meridians and chakras, we can identify emotional states that are body-based and therefore natural in human expression. As we have seen, these natural emotions associated here with chakras and meridians are: joy, empathy, grief, fear, anger, sensuality, personal power, love and surrender. Human experience naturally weaves among these feelings as we respond to life events. They enrich our experience; they teach us to develop greater sensitivity to the human condition. "Unnatural" emotions, such as hate, rage, vengeance, despair, hysteria, etc., which move us toward destruction, are understood as energy distortions or imbalances within the bodymind. Within this energy model of the whole person then we find guidelines for life-promoting and growth-enhancing emotional states.

Emotions can create problems within the bodymind when their expression is seriously imbalanced over a period of time. For example, if they are continuously denied and thus sup-

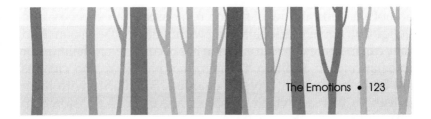

pressed and stored within the body, or if they are over-expressed, emotions can cause energy imbalances which adversely affect health and consciousness. For instance, if anger is felt within the system but consistently denied, its energy will begin to congest within the liver meridian. Conversely, if anger is express excessively, as a kind of broken-tape habit, it can also adversely affect the liver energy.

Through balancing work in the body's energy systems, emotions will automatically, and organically, begin to come into natural expression. Old emotional patterns that no longer serve growth can gradually release form the bodymind.

When emotions are freed from the bindings of familial and collective conditioning, they can be felt, and followed, naturally from within. Awareness and expression of emotions then arise congruently from the body. It is safe to follow their natural wave flow because feelings have been reclaimed and are now "owned" within the individual body. Such body-based, congruent emotions can be trusted as extremely valuable components of wholistic consciousness.

Summary

Emotions have been defined as electrochemical wave motions through the body which provoke visceral, conscious and behavioral changes. I have proposed that the Eastern energy perspectives of meridians and chakras provide a complete map of natural emotions that are related to physiological effects. Those emotions have been described according to their associations with the five elements, meridians and chakras. We have seen that each emotional cluster has a balanced state as well as exaggerated or imbalanced expressions.

The energy maps of the body provide a matrix for identifying, processing and harmonizing emotions. They help us to accept the natural flow of feeling responses as a necessary, and delightful, homeostatic balancing within the whole system. And they can indicate when an emotion has become overwhelming or imbalancing. In addition, the meridian pathways and chakras are body locators for types of emotion. Familiarity with them assists us to read which emotions are most likely stored in different parts of the body.

Body armor can develop as a result of an emotional charge that is held, unexpressed, in the body. The armored body is then limited to those emotional patterns that are fixated within it. The free body, in which armor and energy flows are released, is capable of a wide range of emotional expression and it enjoys the sensitivity and vitality that emotion stimulates. Emotional health is described as a condition in which all emotions can be felt in the body, accepted and expressed in ways that bring greater awareness, freedom and growth.

CHAPTER FIVE

THE MIND

The mind was defined in Chapter One as the observed effects of intellectual, unconscious, superconscious and intuitive functions. Since its inception, psychology has studied the mind extensively, differentiated many mental faculties, devised means of testing them, and generated learning theories which have furthered mental education. We have learned a great deal about developing the intellect and yet we know that we have vast untapped mental capacities. For example, the "higher" mental faculties associated with spiritual development are not so well known. Parapsychology has investigated extra-sensory abilities and yet many of the faculties and feats reported by mentalists or mystics are little understood. The energy maps of meridians and chakras provide definition for many of these faculties; they also give us a matrix for a developmental progression of consciousness.

In this chapter we will be considering those mental faculties which are associated with the energy systems of the body. They are innate, if not all realized, faculties by virtue of their provision through the natural law of the energy pathways and centers.

Conscious and Unconscious Minds

Energy permeates both conscious and unconscious minds. In fact it may provide one of the most valuable bridges between the two. For example, when meridians and/or chakras are affected on the body, unconscious material (usually related to the issues associated with the particular energy meridian or chakra) can directly issue up to consciousness in the moment. Also, a person who has recently received an acupuncture or acupressure session normally reports vivid dreaming, suggesting that when energy is opened in a part of the body that had previously been congested, unconscious material may be brought closer to the surface of consciousness. A poetic dream catalog was given in the *Nei Ching* which contains general guidelines for determining which of the 12 organ meridians is associated with a particular dream motif, suggesting that the ancient Chinese understood a familiar relationship with the dreaming (unconscious) process and energy flow.

Just as body armor tends to fix certain emotional complexes into the body and thus limit emotional expression toward those complexes, mental programs from conditioning are fixed into neural patterns in the brain and nervous system. These basic programs of the mind are derived from very early familial conditioning, socialization within the culture and education. They include introjected directives from parents, belief systems and early primal decisions about life made as a result of emotion-filled experience. They form the core and metaprogram patterns that are principally unconscious. In popular psychology such patterns are called "old tapes" to denote their persevering quality once they are activated. They exert a powerful mental influence on thinking and behavior from an unconscious level. Energy flow through such repressed patterns can bring them into con-

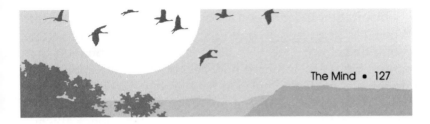

sciousness where they can be reevaluated and changed when appropriate.

Right and Left Brains

During the scientific age left brain functions—linear thought, logic, mathematics, verbal constructions—have been strongly emphasized, while right brain functions—symbolic thought, imaging, creative thinking, spatial relationships—have been somewhat neglected. Both brains are critical to a holographic perspective and their coordinative unity seems important.

The midline energy pathway of the Governing Vessel helps to unify right and left brains. It travels directly over the corpus collusum, a nerve bundle that connects the two brains. One branch of this meridian travels from outside the head straight into the center of the brain. When the meridian is open and energized, it feeds and helps to unify left and right hemispheres of the brain. Clearing and activating this meridian brings a sense of centeredness, unity of consciousness and clarity.

The Five Elements and Mental Faculties

In the following section, mental faculties associated with the five elements and their related meridians will be described. Each of these faculties is inherently available in some measure to all people, regardless of intelligence level. Yet some are developed while others lie dormant. By assessing the energy support associated with these various faculties we can often find ways to enhance their development.

THE ELEMENT FIRE:
INSPIRATION, INTUITION AND DISCRIMINATION

Inspiration, intuition and discrimination are mental processes associated with the fire element, its organs and attendant energy pathways.

Inspiration and intuition are believed to arise from the heart. When the heart and its meridian are open, one can receive promptings from one's own heart (spirit) and inspiration from nature. Similarly, intuitive hunches, insights and impressions are readily available. Intuition may become blocked when the fire element is low and its energy congested. Mental faculties are impaired and there is a scattered quality in the mind. Kaptchuk describes this state:

> When Shen (heart spirit) loses its harmony, the individual's eyes may lack luster and his thinking may be muddled. A person so affected may be slow and forgetful, or perhaps suffer from insomnia. Certain Shen disharmonies are marked by unreasonable responses to the environment, such as incoherent speech. Extreme Shen disharmony can lead to unconsciousness or violent madness. (The Web That Has No Weaver, 1983)

A student described his experience of opening his heart and discovering increased mental inspiration in the following way: "A flame exploded in my heart as an answer to some of my life questions. As I go in this direction I am experiencing an increasing joy that is impossible to contain."

Mental discrimination also involves the fire element. The small intestine meridian, mate of the heart, is said to give the ability to "sort the pure from the impure." In digestion, of course, this is the process of separating nutrients from waste material. The parallel mental ability is that of being able to sort out the useful, true, or "pure" data from what is false, or "waste."

Discernment has been associated with heart knowing in the Christian tradition and is known to be bestowed on a person through spiritual practice. Discrimination and discernment can be strengthened through energy work on the small intestine meridian.

THE EARTH ELEMENT: REFLECTION

Reflection is associated with the earth element, which involves the spleen (pancreas) and stomach meridians. Reflection is the process of going over data in the mind after the event. It includes the ability to learn from mistakes, and to remain conscious and grounded (reality-based) in the face of unpleasant thoughts or feelings. When earth energy is balanced, reflection can be a valuable mental process for examining old data stored

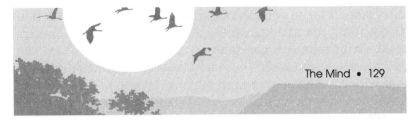

in the mind, and updating it with current reality. However, when this energy is imbalanced, reflection can turn into obsessive going over and over the same material without progression or resolution. Such cyclic thinking can become dogmatism over time.

The earth element is also associated with taking in nourishment, including mental "food," and "digesting" or absorbing it. If the element is balanced this food will nourish mental life appropriately and be replaced by new food. But imbalance causes one to "chew and chew" on the same data, ideas and belief systems, with little or no consideration for whether or not the process is nurturing. This is the essence of "obsessive" thinking.

Of all the energetic associations, this one most closely expresses the "monkey mind"—what Buddhists call the flighty nature of mind—which the meditator must confront and overcome. The thinking circulates in the head, with little reference to sensations and feelings in the body, or the stabilizing reality of the ground beneath the feet.

The great downward sweep of the stomach meridian provides a grounding stream. When this meridian is open and free, it helps to connect thinking with impressions from the body and external realities of the environment. There is a direct connection between physiological processes of the organs and the mind. The circuits of the bodymind are open. Thus the thinker is able to integrate the truth of the whole body.

THE METAL ELEMENT: STRUCTURE

The metal element, represented by the lung and large intestine meridians, supports structure in thinking. The mental functions supported by metal apply to bringing space ("heaven," or spiritual realities) into physical form, or formulating the abstractions that bridge space and form. Creating theories and deriving the rules and laws that support them are metal functions.

The two meridians provide a model for the ebb and flow of

energy and life, through the rhythmic inhalation/exhalation of breath (lung meridian), and the assimilation/elimination processes (large intestine meridian). Applied to the mind the model describes how we take in "heavenly" energy (direct communication with the cosmos) through the breath; give it structure and meaning with our thinking; and "exhale" or discard what we cannot use.

A spiritual quality is inherent in the metal element. The lung meridian is sometimes called "the priest of the temple," or the "official" who receives the pure chi from heaven. This inner priest or priestess can bring guidance based on cosmic order from "heaven," beyond dogma and beyond the limits of the ego. Before the priest is realized, thought structure is based on parental conditioning, or dogma and philosophies encountered in life. But when breath has been fully claimed as one's own the inner priest is activated. The breath then flows naturally with a full in-breath (taking in, receiving from heaven), followed by a full out-breath (letting go, releasing back to the cosmos), and the cycle begins again without interruption. One rides with the Tao.

Unobstructed metal energy assists flowing with the ever-changing reality of the Tao. We can theorize about It, and let those theories go, knowing they are always only approximations of It. We can create temporary structures and let them go when they no longer serve. We can gain momentary enlightenment and let it go when, in the next moment, we are presented with another incomprehensible aspect of It. Thus, the true priest will be humble before the Tao, knowing his own mind, complex and magnificent though it may be, is not capable of fathoming the whole tapestry of Tao.

When the metal energy is out of balance, however, the mind will tend to create structures, theories and rigid belief systems which it will hang on to and worry about long after they have ceased to match reality. The person imbalanced in metal can live in an abstract world of his own, full of fantasies, old worn-out beliefs, and especially old sorrows (see Emotions), that have little to do with the real environment or other people. One can become dogmatic, aloof and deluded.

The large intestine meridian has been called the "janitor within the temple" or "the dust bin collector." The mental function of cleaning out old ideas, outdated data, outmoded beliefs is

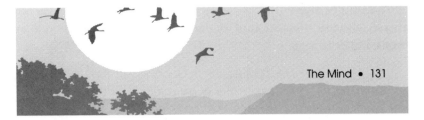

controlled by this meridian which runs up through the neck and into the face. Having a free flow of energy along this meridian greatly assists mental clarity and flexibility. It helps to keep thinking consistent with present data and reality instead.

THE WATER ELEMENT: THE BRAIN AND THE WILL

The water element, expressed in the bladder and kidney meridians, is said to feed the brain in the Chinese system. It is associated with bones and marrow and the brain is called the "sea of marrow." According to the *Nei Ching*, the kidneys store the vital physical energy which feeds the brain; both bladder and kidney meridians send internal branches of energy directly into it. Since the brain is the primary seat of mental activity, its nourishment is crucial for clear thinking.

It is amazing to observe that when a person's kidney energy is low, thinking is often scattered and mental concentration low. The mind may be flooded with fearful thoughts and feelings which can preoccupy the person completely and prevent effective reasoning. When the kidney energy is strengthened the person will experience an increase in mental clarity and stamina. Events or thoughts that previously has seemed overwhelming can be handled with confidence. As we saw in Chapter Four, fear is the predominant emotion for a person with low kidney energy. Fear is a paralyzer of thinking. I have found many times that a person is not able to cope, mentally or socially, until the kidney energy is strengthened.

Will power is traditionally associated with the water element. Connelly says in her book, *Traditional Acupuncture: The Law of the Five Elements:* "The force propelling a person toward actually doing something comes from the clarity within the water element." Part of that force is the quality of will, one of the most necessary mental attributes for a conscious and productive life.

Assagioli devoted an entire book, *The Act of Will* (1971), to the cultivation of the will. He claimed that conscious will was an absolutely essential function for awakening into higher development. He said:

At a given moment, perhaps during a crisis, one has a vivid and unmistakable inner experience of the (will's) reality and nature. When danger threatens to paralyze us, suddenly, from the mysterious depths of our being, surges an unsuspected strength which enables us to place a firm foot on the edge of the precipice or confront an aggressor....(One is) endowed with the power to choose, to relate, to bring about changes in his own personality, in others, in circumstances.

This surge of unsuspected strength accurately describes the rise of stored energy from the kidney energy.

THE WOOD ELEMENT: PLANNING, DECIDING AND JUDGMENT

The wood element governs those creative processes that have to do with vision, planning, making decisions and judgments, and implementing projects. The liver meridian is related to vision at all levels, from seeing clearly the environment around us with the physical eyes to internal, spiritual vision. In fact, the liver is said to be the seat of the soul in the *Nei Ching:* "The liver harbors the soul and the spiritual faculties." Thus it can be associated with overall direction and purpose in life. It also supports the ability to plan the incremental steps required to manifest visions and purpose. When liver energy is strong and balanced one has the mental capacity to generate short-and long-term goals and to strike a direction in life that is appropriate to one's own spiritual purpose.

The liver's mate, the gall bladder, gives the ability to make decisions and implement plans. It also facilitates "right" judgment, that is, the faculty of assessing appropriate alternatives which preserve integrity of the system. The two meridians together provide the most basic components of the creative process—vision and actualization. At the most fundamental level they facilitate the realization of true purpose in life.

A case of strong wood imbalance in a client exemplifies the progression that can occur when this energy is cleared. A man came to my classes who was aimless and fairly depressed even though he was basically strong, young and intelligent. He had no direction in life, couldn't decide where to live, or what work (if any) he should do. He had a bad case of hepatitis a few years earlier and was a serious marijuana user (both are injurious to the liver). After the hepatitis he had suffered a "black depression" for several months and complained that since then he had no meaning in his life. When the depression recurred he would use marijuana to avoid it, which only made his condition worse.

When I started working with him as a client he became even more depressed simply because he became more aware of his actual situation in life. But gradually he began to make simple decisions—he fixed his car so he could travel, and cleaned up his carpentry tools in case he should decide to use them. After several classes and sessions he decided to move to another city. Once there he decided to follow up on our work by seeing a Taoist master acupuncturist who continued the work of balancing the wood element. Over the next year he began to take hold of his life. He went to work with his tools, remodeling his room, found a spiritual teacher, began to meditate, met a loving and steady professional woman whom he eventually married. During this time he gave up marijuana completely in favor of meditation. Now he and his wife have bought a home, he has his own small construction company and definitely has direction and meaning in life.

Mental Functions and the Chakras

Just as we can use the energy map of the chakra system to trace physical development, we can use it to differentiate natural mental functions and to trace development of consciousness, from the most primitive to the most enlightened.

THE ROOT CHAKRA: SURVIVAL INSTINCTS

The root chakra is associated with the most rudimentary survival instincts which have been described as "jungle mentality." Fear of attack and insecurity about physical survival are common reactions associated with this chakra. Recognizing pain quickly in the body, being aware of environmental threats and protecting oneself are skills related to the root. When a person has his energy centered here, he will be concerned about being attacked or hurt by others. The level of awareness is often compared to animal instincts—wariness, intense perception of physical details, quick attention to environmental threats and procreative drives that are specifically biological. There is sharp attunement with nature and animals, and a strong sensation function. These instinctual functions are especially valuable for surviving in a physical body. The person who has a strong root chakra, usually by virtue of secure development in the first seven years, will be grounded in physical reality and have a strong sense of his capacity to take care of himself physically.

THE SECOND CHAKRA: SENSUALITY AND CREATIVITY

The second chakra, located close to the genital organs, is principally related to sensuality and sexuality, as distinguished from the more primitive procreative drives linked with the root chakra. Through sensuality the sensate functions are developed as one pays attention to, and appreciates physical and material sensations.

The energy of the second chakra is very powerful; it is here that the vital physical essence (of the water element) is stored. This essence can be expressed automatically, through natural sexuality. Or it can be contained and shaped to create through volition. For example, this center is termed the "hara" in Oriental martial and healing arts, which practice building and storing energy here that can be called upon at will, and focused through mental concentration, to accomplish extraordinary physical and/or healing acts. The practice of saving and raising second chakra energy to higher chakras where it can be applied for purposes other than sexuality is used in some forms of yoga. However, to habitually suppress or sublimate this energy is psychologically risky since much unconscious material can collect here. The yogi Satyananda, as reported by Motoyama, has identified the unconscious with this chakra, and in particular the collective unconscious.

THE THIRD CHAKRA: EGO STRUCTURE, REASON AND LOGIC

The third chakra could be called the center of the "biocomputer"; it is associated with the mental abilities of reason and logic that can process data received through the regular (as distinct from "extra") senses. These abilities can be trained to a high level of development. Valid reasoning, or logic, is the skill of drawing reasonable inferences from digital data. Through reasoning one is able to think through, and create structure for, vast amounts of bits of data. With sufficient accurate data, reasoning results in reality-based conclusions; if data is limited, or false, inferences can still be logical, but untrue.

The third chakra is sometimes referred to also as the "emotional brain." This has reference to the tendency in people who are not developed in reason and logic to be run by emotions. As we saw in Chapter Four, most emotions arise within this center of the body, thus they have compelling power within or around this chakra. Also, when ego strength and boundaries are not well formed, it is common for one to "pick up" emotions from others in this center.

The third chakra is the center most extensively related to personal ego. At this literal "gut" level of consciousness one tends to orient toward personal interest and personal power. During the developmental state when this center predominates— ages 14 to 21—personal identity is shaped. As the adolescent attempts to define himself he tends to see other people, and the world in general, through the lens of his own history, needs and feelings. He is appropriately "ego-centric" during this time, and relates to life in general based on his own sensory and emotional comfort. He learns to assert himself and his own power to get what he needs, and in doing so, gains self-confidence and a certain self-security. Ego is firmly rooted and can act as the stabilizing self-reference center for survival in the world.

At the opposite extreme, of course, is the person who is underdeveloped in this center. He may suffer from inadequate ego development and thus exhibit an "inferiority complex," which can cause a constant search outside of himself for ego support from others.

It would seem that third chakra consciousness is fairly well developed at the upper educational levels in the Western world. The physical self-preservation (and self-destruction) technology we have developed, the ways in which we have harnessed nature to serve ourselves—these feats are remarkable examples of linear reason. In fact, it is probably possible for a person to be very successful and reach high achievement in the contemporary world, through development within the first three chakras only.

Western psychology, from Freud through ego psychology, has emphasized the importance of the perspective and skills related to this chakra. It has taught the importance of a pragmatic consciousness with an intellectual, rational framework to organize behavior in expedient and serviceable way in order to function in the external world. Developed rationality, as exhibited in genuinely cultured and educated people, is held as the epitome of human development.

The industrial and scientific revolutions are, in some measure, the result of the flowering of reason. Through reason and logic we have also constructed machines (computers) which can now carry out some of these functions better and faster than we can. Yet many contemporary philosophers, psychologists and social analysts believe that we have reached the outer limits of human advancement through data collection, analysis, and technology. Destructive teachnical potential, environmental exploitation, and reduction of earth resources threaten our very survival. Many of our serious human problems remain unsolved.

From an Eastern perspective, however, third chakra cultivation is viewed as an essential base for further growth in consciousness through the higher chakras. For example, when mental functions are limited in the adult to the third chakra, the abilities of reason, logic and personal power tend to focus on individual security, physical and psychological comfort. But when they serve as a foundation for the development of higher consciousness, they can lend strength and precision to execute visions of health and well-being for all sentient beings.

THE FOURTH CHAKRA: INTEGRATION AND EMPATHY

The fourth through seventh chakras have been termed the

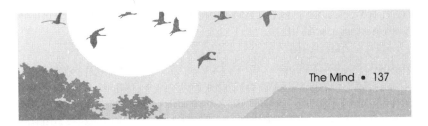

"higher" chakras to denote the transcendent states of conscious-ness available through them. Development within these chakras is not common; we must search spiritual literature to find ex-amples of saints, teachers and yogis who have actualized qualities of the upper chakras. Here spiritual development can begin to merge with, and eventually take precedence over, psychological work. A number of contemporary teachers believe that raising consciousness into these centers is crucial for planetary survival.

The fourth, or heart, chakra is associated with the integration of the "higher" and "lower" aspects of human consciousness. It is here that individual drives for self-preservation, ego and power, held in the first three chakras, begin to integrate with the capacity for transcendent consciousness available through the upper four chakras.

The capacity for empathy is developed in the heart. The ability to put oneself in others' shoes, rather than judge them from one's own ego perspective, enables a person to extend sensitivity and help to others. This extension of awareness be-yond ego leads to the ability to both give and receive love, without addiction or attachment. Ultimately one can develop the capacity for unconditional love through the fourth chakra. The realm of the extra-senses becomes accessible here. Sensing with the heart, a kind of feeling intuition, makes it possible for a person to feel what is behind the words, circumstances or actions of another person. Discrimination, or discernment, develops as an ability to integrate both mental analysis of data with felt wholistic information.

Individual conscience, an inner knowing of what is right, life-promoting, and not harmful to others, arises through this chakra. This ability is distinct form the social conscience developed through outer training, religion or philosophy, or the expedience of "enlightened self-interest." Rather, it is a prompting from within the Self, toward right action that includes consideration of the oneness of all life.

The capacity to forgive—oneself as well as others—arises within the heart chakra. In his book, *Joy's Way*, Brugh Joy claims that the ability to forgive allows a person to "move from the law of karma (action and reaction) into the law of grace." In the same book he teaches how hurts of the past can be dissolved within the energy of the heart chakra. In psychological work this method can circumvent an enormous amount of analytical process in which every trauma is brought to consciousness and worked through at a cognitive level.

In this mental stage of development the greater whole of life comes into perspective. An influx of divine energy meets the open heart, bringing with it a direct experience of an order and grace beyond ego. Out of this knowing, one is able to surrender personal ego capacities and powers over to that transcendent order, and to enter the greater flow of divine direction.

THE FIFTH CHAKRA:
CREATIVITY AND TRANSCENDENT ALIGNMENT

The fifth or throat chakra focuses the auditory function. This includes all abilities associated with hearing and sounding, including the faculty of processing information through language in all its aspects—hearing, reading, thinking and speaking. Much of our education relies on and promotes this faculty. We learn to hear, understand, read and speak words. Consequently in most educated people auditory learning is developed and comprehension through language is favored. Understanding language is the first step toward more complex operations such as analyzing data, building concepts and engaging in reasoning. Non-word utterances, such as toning, singing and chanting are also centered here. Truth from the individual spirit of the heart naturally arises into the throat through speech and singing when that spirit is liberated.

The fifth (throat) chakra is also associated with creativity and receiving transcendent reality. Creativity originates in the procreative drive of the second chakra and it progresses through the throat chakra in the production of refined artistic works and/or verbal power. When this chakra is fully developed a person may become a co-creator with the divine. Rama, Ballentine and Ajaya describe this process as follows:

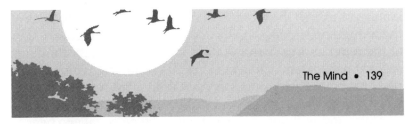

In a certain psychological sense one's words, his utterances, create the universe within which he exists. The throat chakra is the focus of vocalization and singing, verbalization and creativity... Through the repetition of verbal ritual, one's reality can be restructured and recreated. New words and new thought create a new world. (Yoga and Psychotherapy, 1976)

The reactive and chaotic impulses of the lower chakras no longer dominate consciousness when one gains mastery in the fifth chakra. Rather, a person can create what he wants, through the power of mental concentration and will, and with the wisdom of transcendent guidance. Swami Radha describes this as a process of giving power to the inner voice:

When the "voice of the Self" or the still, small voice within is heard and given attention, recognition and gratitude, the aspirant can be truly said to be in touch with the Higher Self, which is now given back its rightful rulership. When you identify with anything other than your Higher Self, you make a very serious error which at some time you will have to rectify. (Kundalini Yoga for the West, 1978)

Consciousness within this chakra brings the ability to understand symbolism. Archetypal symbols, mythic images and primal signs which can arise from the deep unconscious are often brought out into creative expression. The creative act can thus become a tool for integrative psychological work and expanding consciousness.

The extra-sense of clairaudience opens in the fifth chakra. It is the ability to inwardly hear the truth, through the still, small voice within, or behind another person's external verbalizations. For example, one who has an awakened fifth chakra can hear many truths about another simply through the voice tone.

Through fifth chakra development one learns mental mastery by becoming aware of how constructions of the mind can manifest through the word. Swami Radha says, "The balance of the body, mind and speech, is nearing completion in the awareness of the mind and its manifestation in speech. Straight thinking, straight actions and directness are the results...." Tremendous personal power can result from this ability, but since one is also more attuned to transcendent order, there is a greater understanding and willingness to surrender the personal ego over to that order. Divine guidance, which goes beyond the limits of ego, is available to nurture the soul. Within this chakra one learns to commit oneself to the position of "Thy Will be done."

THE SIXTH CHAKRA: CLAIRVOYANCE AND INTUITION

Through development of the sixth chakra, located in the middle of the forehead, consciousness can become unified (right and left brain working together) and whole. The two spinal energy streams, ida and pingali, which have crisscrossed in duality through the lower five chakras, come together as one in the brow. The eye (and "I") becomes single. One sees oneself as a divine whole Self (yogic literature claims that the true self is met here), which is part of the greater whole of the cosmos. Ramakrishna described his experience of the illuminated sixth chakra as follows:

The supreme Self is directly known and the individual experiences samadhi when the mind comes here. The supreme Self is so near then that it seems as if one is merged in Him, identified with Him. (Ancient Wisdom and Modern Science, Quoted in Grof, 1984)

This chakra is associated with the faculty of comprehending holographically, and swiftly. From here one can instantly realize a whole truth, or gestalt, that might take days to reach through linear logic. It is said that true intelligence is seated here. One can both perceive and generate wholistic mental images and abstract concepts.

Through the brow we acquire the ability to see clearly into the essence of things. This seeing relates to both the physical eyes and the "third eye," the unified clairvoyant eye of the brow, which enables one to perceive the "unseen," beyond constraints of time and space. The unified eye can be focused, like a laser, to see any particular person or subject very deeply. This kind of seeing is called "clairvoyance," which is the ability to see through things,

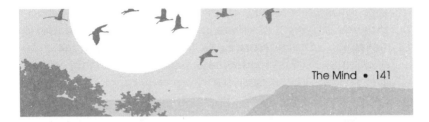

across great distances and backwards and forward in time.

Yoga psychology assigns the faculty of intuition to the sixth chakra. This intuition is different from the feeling intuition of the heart and the fire element mentioned earlier. Intuition of the brow is beyond confusion with emotion and is not influenced by the personal unconscious, nor even the constraints of the physical world. It is more removed from the personal and has a wide reach into the cosmos. The great prophets throughout history, who were able to "see" events far into the future, were focused in the brow chakra. Intuition from this center is strong and clear. Rama, Ballentine and Ajaya describe it as "true intuition."

> True intuition is a stable, reliable function of the higher levels of consciousness and awareness from which a wider range of information is accessible. There intellect and emotion flow together and become integrated, permitting a new kind of knowing, a kind of knowing which both depends on and promotes self-realization. Intuition unquestionably comes from the highest source of consciousness. (Yoga and Psychotherapy, 1976)

Two types of intuition have been delineated within the brow: creative and inward-directed. Creative intuition is the ability to bring superconscious insights into concrete manifestation in the world. Inward-directed intuition gives the capacity of direct knowing about the innermost nature of things, without normal training or collection of data. It is a faculty for tuning into Universal Mind. The guru who knows when his disciple will arrive, without benefit of physical communication, exhibits this ability. Spiritual literature contains many accounts of the "miraculous" (and accurate) knowledge of spiritual teachers who have not studied the specific fields about which they speak.

> The yogi assiduously cultivates the brow through training and practices that will open it to modes of awareness for which we

have potential, but which we are at present not able to imagine. It means escaping the confines of our culturally endorsed, everyday reality. it means escaping the limited concepts of a consciousness which is oriented around material, externally observable phenomena. It means moving beyond the limitations of time, space and causality.

THE SEVENTH CHAKRA: ULTIMATE ATTAINMENT

The seventh, or crown chakra, located at the top of the head, is usually symbolized by a thousand-petaled lotus which represents the almost limitless expansion of which human consciousness is capable. In this center, which is rarely realized fully, the distinction between the personal and the cosmic completely disappears. One experiences "union with the divine," and a state of incomparable bliss. Personal identity, emotions and the ordinary mind are no longer relevant.

Ni Hua Ching has described consciousness of the seventh chakra in his translation of the *Tao Te Ching* as follows:

He unites his mind with the unnameable Subtle Origin of the multi-universe, in which there is no past, no present and no future. This is how an absolute being deals with his mind. (1981)

Those who have experienced a sustained opening within the crown say that it cannot be described in words since it transcends the ordinary mind and language. It has been compared to the light of countless suns, and is said to completely transcend earthly reality. In his book *Cosmic Consciousness*, Bucke described the illuminating expansions of consciousness that Descartes, Blake, Whitman and others received spontaneously, without the formal training that yogis practice to achieve these states. In all cases "cosmic consciousness" permanently changed the subjects. Several, including the philosopher Descartes, had only one such experience, of a minute in duration. Yet that experience provided the sustained inspiration for many ideas and/or creative productions of an elevated nature for many years.

I had a cosmic consciousness experience one day while driving. It lasted less than 15 minutes but seemed like a piece of eternity out of time. It was as if everything were illuminated and I understood, in an instant gestalt, all that I had been studying and contemplating for several years. Great joy accompanied the

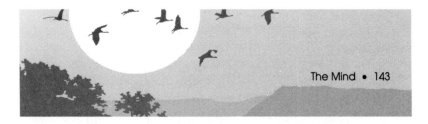

experience, but it was not heart's joy. Rather, it was an ecstasy of comprehension that went far beyond my usual mental capacities. I wrote in my journal, "to open into this now moment opens into all the galaxies—everything is available, all the truth of What Is." At one point I knew that I was enlightened—in that moment. Later I realized that enlightenment was not a permanent state (which I had previously naively imagined), but for me a temporary glimpse of what was actually possible in a body. As I write this, years later, there is still a sense of it in my mind and it affects my entire orientation to life even now.

The soul can leave the physical body through the crown. Some yogis have consciously chosen their time of death through this means. Awareness of the crown can be extremely important in work with dying people because of its potential gateway for the smooth departure of the soul. Motoyama says

> *When the "Gate of Brahman" in this chakra is opened, one can leave the physical body and enter the realms of the astral or the causal (emotional and spiritual). (Science and Evolution of Consciousness, 1978)*

Psycho-Spiritual Work and the Higher Chakras

Traditional psychology has not addressed crown chakra consciousness since it transcends the psyche. Psycho-spiritual work and transpersonal psychology, however, must require knowledge of this center. Rama, Ballentine and Ajaya refer to its importance:

> *Though in a sense this experience (of the crown) lies beyond modern psychology, since it departs from the limitations of the psyche, it is obviously of vital importance....It offers the vantage*

point from which the mind can be most clearly appreciated. It serves as a crucial point of orientation. Though it lies beyond the realm of mental functioning, it provides the key to the framework in which the functioning of the mind becomes intelligible, and all the aspects of experience can be integrated into a unified theory. Furthermore, the nature of this state is so fundamental to the nature of man's being that to be completely successful any psychological theory must at least be compatible to its existence. (Yoga and Psychotherapy, 1976)

I believe it is especially important for transpersonal psychologists to be familiar with the upper chakras (fourth through seventh) even though traditional psychology has focused on the first three. Many of our standards for "normalcy" are based on healthy functioning in the first three chakras with little or no consideration for the others. Some people who have had spiritual emergence experiences through "opening" in the upper chakras have been classified as psychotic and placed in mental wards where they have been kept on drugs and/or convinced by their therapists that their experiences of higher consciousness were false, illusory or pathological.

One of my clients. a highly accomplished professional person, had a cosmic consciousness experience that changed her life. Through it she gained heightened clarity, an opening of the heart chakra into agape love, and a much deeper commitment to her life's work. However, prior to her recognition of the significance of this experience, she spent several days in a psychiatric ward into which she was committed by well-meaning but naive friends who thought she was having a psychotic break. Even after her release from the hospital it took many months to convince her friends that she was stable. Eventually they came to recognize the truth of her spiritual experience, after observing the developmental change in her consciousness and behavior.

As more people see a spiritual life, as larger and larger numbers meditate and engage in other spiritual practices, there will probably be many more experiences like the one described above. Hopefully we will learn to support spiritual emergence, in individuals and in the world, rather than reject it and/or tag it with psychiatric labels. For it is through the development of the higher chakras that we can take the next evolutionary step

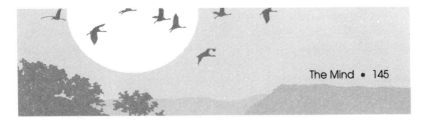

wherein we can achieve true mastery over ourselves and live in harmony with humankind and the environment.

Summary

In this chapter we have explored the mind and its relationships with the energy systems of meridians and chakras. Various mental faculties have been linked with specific energy pathways or centers. It has been shown that the energy maps provide a catalog of mental functions which are natural and attainable, from the most primitive or simplistic through the most advance stages of consciousness.

This full range of mental capability, combined with emotions and sensations from the body, and undergirded by knowing of the soul, brings the capacity for whole being consciousness. Motoyama has called it a unified totality of consciousness. He says:

> Consciousness has enormous potential. It can—and unconsciously does—link up directly with other minds and universal forms. It need not be bound by the five senses, by time, nor by space. As mystics have long held, consciousness is a unified totality; the divisive limits that we experience in everyday life are ultimately illusions. (*Science and Evolution of Consciousness*, 1978)

Such a state of awareness goes far beyond the intellect, or any other single faculty. Whole being consciousness places one within the synchronistic flow of the Great Order.

CHAPTER SIX

RETURNING TO SOUL

A Vision of Wholeness

Now that we have looked in detail at the parts of the whole person, it is important to bring them together to understand how they interact as a multi-faceted system. In this chapter we will consider the possible human development that leads to wholeness, individuation and a return to the soul as the master of destiny.

In this era of wholistic thinking we recognize that the mind can no longer be isolated in function from the body, that emotions influence our thinking and that the body's ills can often be traced back to our neurotic tendencies. Yet we still take our ill bodies to medical practitioners, our psychological problems to psychiatrists and psychologists and our spiritual unrests to the church. We fragment our views of ourselves and employ therapeutic approaches that address only one part of the system without reference to the whole. We know, of course, that we are whole persons, and yet we tend to act as if we were at one time a body, another a mind or an emotion. Sometimes we think of ourselves as our roles— mother, brother, lawyer, teacher. Sometimes we identify with any one or a number of psychological or physical labels that momentarily describe a part of us. Is a whole person in fact, simply a collection of thousands of characteristics? You might ask, "If I were living from the whole of me, what would I be like?" Through my work with people I have come to understand a whole person as one who has vitality, awareness and development in body, mind, emotions and soul, and in whom these seemingly separate factors integrate and cooperate in a harmonic progression toward soul realization or destiny.

If we are to realize ourselves as whole, individual beings, it seems necessary to follow and reclaim all parts of ourselves. In psychological terms this means we need to recognize and integrate the truths that arise from the body, the mind, the emotions and the soul as we individuate. It means a new kind of self-work and a new kind of psychotherapy. It means viewing a person from a wellness model rather than from the traditional disease or neurosis models. It means being able to work at both personality and soul levels. How would such work proceed? Where would it lead? What methods are needed to carry it forward? In this chapter we will consider these questions and investigate how psycho-spiritual work can facilitate wholeness.

Individuation: A Psycho-Spiritual Process

At the core of all wisdom teachings throughout history, spiritual or philosophical, East and West, is the counsel: "Know thyself." After the student has penetrated any true system, belief or teaching, he is directed to the "kingdom within" his own soul, where the truth and meaning of his existence is ultimately held.

Individuation is a learning process of recovering the soul and liberating the body and consciousness to follow its destiny. Jung taught that individuation was the final, and most important, unfoldment in life. He thought this phase of development could most appropriately be accomplished in the second half of life, when there was enough maturity, life experience and the presence of death to urge it forward. Arnold Mindell has found that dying people are often willing to break through many of the limitations that have run their lives to become their true selves in the days or hours before death. I believe individuation can occur before those last hours, and even before midlife, in our time. I have known many aspirants who, still in the first half of their lives, are well on their way. I believe there are many old souls in incarnation at this time, and that the pressures of our planetary problems help to awaken them to their true purposes. Further, we now have more effective psycho-physical technologies for liberating the body and consciousness than in the past.

The process of individuation can unfold through many different avenues. Some come to themselves through pursuing the activity and work that really have meaning for them. Creative people, no matter what the medium, often discover their souls within the heart of their creative process. Others find the self through committed spiritual practice. Still others arrive at it through a continuous learning and growing process that can happen within any field. And some come to it through their own introspection over time. Personal therapy is one of the avenues that can be helpful, especially when it empowers the person and teaches her how to follow all of herself.

In Chapter One the distinction between personality and soul was delineated. The soul carries the spiritual essence and purpose of the individual person. The personality, on the other hand, is a product of societal and family conditioning, formed to adapt to prevailing collective values. As long as a person is completely dominated by his personality (or the personalities of others), he is usually more attuned to collective expectations than to fulfilling his own individual path in life. He is often driven by specific directives or the unfulfilled dreams of his parents, for example. To discover his own inherent nature, his own soul and his own direction, and to follow them to actualization is a different process altogether. Finding the true self and bringing it forth into life requires psycho-spiritual development.

In Transpersonal Integration we wish to empower the soul as an active factor in the process of individuation and also to empower its specific purpose. Personality work, which is primarily psycho-physical, is focused within the context of assisting that empowerment. Where the personality has covered over and obstructed realization of the self it can be examined and restructured. Spiritual work, or soul attunement, can unfold as the personality is freed.

Phases of Individuation

1. SETTING AN INTENTION

The first act toward individuation is the desire to live from one's Self and the intention to find and follow that Self. *It is a creative act that initiates a creative process rather than a problem-solving one.* The decision to follow one's Self can come late in life, after many unsatisfying directions have already been explored, or it can be made early when visions and dreams of life are fresh. This decision alone can mobilize all parts of a person toward self-realization, and a process of inner direction can begin to unfold. For example, some of the adolescents I taught had strong dreams and attractions toward particular work or life purposes. I urged them to hold to and develop their ideas even when they seemed far removed from what was going on in the culture at that time. When they are honored, dreams can be powerful magnets that draw us toward their realization. Some of these students later developed completely new work and lifestyles through believing in and following their dreams.

When a person first comes to work with me I suggest placing our work together within the context of self-realization; when it seems appropriate we may align both of our souls to that task from the beginning. This orientation signals to the unconscious and the deep self that we wish to respect the truth of the whole being and that we are even seeking help from those deep levels. I certainly accept and respect the problems or symptoms the person may bring to solve. But at the same time I also encourage her to gain a wider view and to look beneath the problems to find what she actually wants to create in life. Solving problems can confine the work within the limited range of the problem; we want to access the greater potential of the whole person. Jung once said that we do not ever solve problems, we simply outgrow them (because we grow into a larger perspective).

2. RECLAIMING AWARENESS IN ALL PARTS OF ONESELF

The resources for individuation all lie within the person, specifically within the meaningful signals that are received continuously from the body, mind, feelings, as well as the intuitive and spiritual faculties. When a person knows how to read and follow those signals she will be able to follow her own truth. As we have seen, however, a person is seldom aware of all these parts, much less their signals. Thus, she does not have access to the whole of her own information. In fact, sometimes she may be completely cut off from an entire part. It is common for a person to have virtually no access to the body or the feelings for instance.

Important first learning tasks, therefore, are those of reconnecting with all the parts of oneself and discovering how to follow signals from all those parts. With these skills in place a person will have access to multiple inner resources. She will be able to follow herself authentically through later more complex work in the personality, as well as for soul attunement.

Regaining contact and awareness within the body and learning how to process its signals are fundamental skills for both health and individuation. Yet these natural abilities have often been lost by adulthood. Many people who come to me with distressing physical symptoms have little or no awareness of their felt body sense. They know they have severe headaches or pains in the shoulder or repeated stomach aches, but when I ask them, with hands on the body, "What are you aware of here, or here?" they answer, "Oh nothing, I don't feel anything."

A high-level executive came to see me about head and neck aches that were becoming so severe they were interfering with his work. He had a band of hard armoring almost an inch thick that began at the base of his head and extended down into the neck. This normally soft tissue felt like bone. As I worked into the armoring during our first session I asked him what he felt. "Nothing," he replied. I was amazed, since this is usually a sensitive area to most people. This man had been cut off from his feelings for a long time. He took the brunt of his stressful work into his body and held it down rather than voice his discomforts, disappointments or vulnerable feelings. Now his body was crying out through headaches. It took an acute body symptom to finally gain his attention because he had disconnected from his body awareness. As we worked together over time, the armor began to release, he regained feeling in the tissue and learned how to pay attention to his body needs before they progressed into symptoms.

Body awareness can be cultivated within each body part. One can relearn (for we all had this awareness in childhood) how to instantaneously notice sensations within the body and then follow them specifically as they move and change. As a person gains body awareness he will be able to quickly pay attention to body signals, find out what the body needs and take care of it, averting conditions that may eventually develop into sickness.

In addition to the health benefits of body awareness, the body contains physiological wisdom and, as we have seen in Chapter Three, the individual's personal history. Both of these invaluable data stores become available by developing body sensitivity.

Many people are also disconnected from their feelings. As we saw in Chapter Four, childhood feelings that were disallowed, or simply too painful to endure, were pushed down and held in the body and cut off from awareness. By adulthood the person no longer has access to feelings of fear, anger, vulnerability or love. Such a person responds to life through thinking alone. If you ask, "How do you feel about this thing or that person?" the answer will usually be an automatic "Nothing." For example, I once asked a woman who had been abused, verbally and sexually, by her father how she felt about him. "I don't feel anything about him," she replied disdainfully. In actual fact, as we explored that relationship more deeply, her inner child was full of feelings about him—rage, sorrow, fear, love and longing.

It is very common for the abused child to disconnect from all feeling and learn to function in life as a thinking machine. This strategy gets the person successfully through the mechanics of life. However, it usually prevents her from going deeper into the well of her own knowing, which must include the wisdom of feeling. It also prevents her from developing satisfying relationships, which always require feeling.

It is also fairly common for people to be disconnected from their own minds and intuitive faculties. Our educational system is predominantly set up to emphasize the accumulation of data within the constraints of prevailing systems and theories. We are programmed to accept and operate from these data bases. Independent thinking and creativity are not only not taught; they are actively discouraged, according to many current studies. Intuitive processes, outside the structure of reason and logic, are not greatly valued. After, or during, formal education a sorting process is usually required to determine what is true from what is not true. Beyond that discernment a person can begin to discover her own thinking and intuitive insights within, or distinct from, her education. A very intelligent 30-year-old once told me she had no ideas of her own apart from the gifted teacher she followed.

Psychotherapy usually does a good job in helping a person to "reality-check" his data bases and to clarify and refine his own thinking processes. The process can also be done alone, however, when a person has the determination and vision to pursue it.

One client of mine had accomplished this task in an unusual way through a process of continual learning. He had grown up in a small town as part of a large family with a very limited outlook and little education. The parents taught by criticism and punishment. He had no other models to show him greater possibilities. By the time he finished high school, he was not confident about his own abilities and had no prospects for life except to work in the local gas station, which he did, for a time. But he felt there must be more to his life. He also felt no support from his family nor community. He decided to move on, to enroll in a school in another, larger community. As he saw a wider perspective, in school and within the new community, he gradually gained a belief in himself and his abilities. He succeeded at his work and kept studying. Next he moved to an even bigger city where there were more school and work opportunities. He kept learning and advancing. Eventually he moved to San Francisco ("I couldn't move to the big city in one leap," he told me) and into a large university, where there were many resources to support his blossoming individuality and career. By the time he saw me he felt he had grown far beyond his parents. He was his own man, in charge of his own mind and charting his own journey.

The spiritual nature and faculties are even more rarely cultivated in our culture than body awareness, feelings or mental abilities. Many people have some knowledge of religious teachings and rituals, and may attend church regularly. But the inner knowing of spiritual truths, and the promptings of the "still wise voice within" are less known. Usually these abilities develop through meditative or contemplative practices over time. They require quiet time, a serious attention to the most subtle inner signs, and often, a closeness to nature. In Transpersonal Integration we encourage the development of spiritual awareness by respecting all of the quiet promptings from within, taking them seriously and urging follow up through development in contemplation or meditation and eventual action

By the time a person is connected with his own awareness, and has occupied body, feelings, mind and spiritual faculties, he has much greater power and a new sense of his broad potential as a whole person. He has seen through some of the other-imposed restrictions that have held him back from that potential, and has probably adjusted his self-concept and many of his goals accordingly. Like the man who finally moved to San Francisco, he is moving on in a more self-directed and fresh way with the life he wants to live rather than the one he inherited. He knows how to follow himself. This person may be able to go full speed ahead, with his awareness as the only necessary ally.

3. Personality Work

Some people move forward nicely with self-directed growth. They choose a direction, set goals, and gather the necessary information and skills to manifest those goals. They succeed in

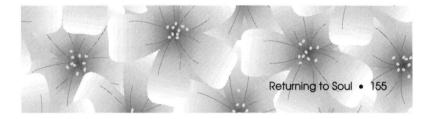

life, work and relationships through progressive steps, making mistakes and correcting their course accordingly. But there may be times when they hit a snag that seems to throw them back into old destructive and self-defeating feelings and behaviors from the past. Irrational insecurity, depression, loneliness or confusion may crop up when there seems to be no reason in the present. Or a person might find himself tangled up in the same kind of problem repeatedly.

Such crises are often brought on by some limiting pattern within the personality that was set in place long ago. Sometimes such patterns happen in response to a great outer shock, like death or natural disaster, which disorients or devastates a person. When ongoing development is curbed by traumatic effects from past history, or shocks in the present, personality work can be very helpful in clearing up those effects. In fact, a time of crisis can provide the most fruitful opportunity for growth because we are then necessarily open to change and new perspectives. During and after the great earthquake of 1989 in northern California, many people took stock of the meaning and purpose of their lives and some made major changes for the better.

UNDERSTANDING THE PERSONALITY

As we saw in Chapter One, the material of the personality and personal psychology derives from the personal history of the current lifetime. Understanding the personality is a psychological process, although it doesn't necessarily require the help of a psychotherapist. A person can explore her own personality alone, through introspection, self analysis, or intimate, honest communication with a friend, although it is often difficult to penetrate through one's own blind spots. Understanding can also be greatly assisted by various psychological theories and techniques, including defined self-help methods and psychotherapy. Traditional psychotherapy seeks to understand personality and behavior primarily through mental observation, reflection and analysis of personal history in discussion between therapist and client. However, many present psychological perspectives tend to label the person according to psychoses, neuroses or at least neurotic tendencies, which is not always growth-promoting.

An understanding of the personality will emerge as the personal history and psychology are examined. Appropriate psychological methods can help bring the light of consciousness into those events, relationships and patterns that have hitherto been "dark," or unconscious. Obvious disturbances, neurotic patterns and self-destructive tendencies which manifest in the mind, emotions or body, must usually be given first attention. Such difficulties often bring a person to therapy in the first place; later they can serve as threads to start an unraveling process within the personality structure that will eventually reveal all its various parts.

Understanding and Processing Personality Through the Body

In addition to psychological methods, integrative bodywork can help to reveal personality structure, since personal history is imprinted within the body. Each body has recorded what actually happened to that person and what psychological effects those events had. I believe that processing, or working through, those effects can be most effectively accomplished through the body.

Transpersonal Integration approaches personality directly through the body. I work with my hands on the client's body as she lies clothed on a table. Simultaneously she and I are also working in consciousness. As I touch various points and parts of her body, I am following the body's energy flow because clearing and balancing the energy as we work promotes security and steadily builds a background harmonic through the whole system. Working this way also deepens the process and gives us easy access to altered states through which we can reach the unconscious.

As a team the client and I uncover the body and personality layers progressively—that is, from surface to deep structures, as the body is ready to reveal them. I follow the client's unfolding process through these layers, trusting her own wholistic wis-

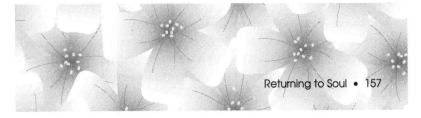

dom, rather than imposing interpretations of my own.

Process Work is particularly effective in understanding and working through personality obstructions in a wholistic way, because it is designed to follow the individual's unique process exactly, with no therapist-designed interpretation or intervention. By following, rather than leading, a person's individual process, we accept the truths that arise simultaneously from body, mind, and emotions and allow them to lead us to the person's own healing and wholeness. Dr. Rachel Remen, who helps people find their own process of health and wholeness, described it well:

> *If I listen to the client, to the essential self of the*
> *other person—the soul, if you like—I find that at*
> *the deepest level of the unconscious mind, the client*
> *knows what's needed....Healing is the very ground of*
> *being. Everything is moving toward wholeness. And*
> *that's all healing is, that movement. Our task is*
> *not to make something happen but to uncover what*
> *is already happening in us and in others, and to*
> *recognize and foster those conditions that nurture it.* (Remen,
> in *Healers on Healing*, 1989)

As we follow a person's own process we can unravel and work through those traumatic or untrue patterns that have impeded her development. The personality can be revealed, and changed where appropriate, at a pace the person can integrate.

Our initial investigations appropriately address the surface structures—the persona and body of personality—which are fairly accessible to conscious observation and reflection, as in traditional psychotherapy. Understanding, and gaining power in, these levels is important so that the person can develop a healthy ego structure from which to function effectively in the world.

The persona, for example, is available for everyone to see. This is the layer of the personality we generally meet in ordinary life, for it represents how the person has chosen to present herself in the world. Beneath that layer we may eventually discover a very different person. But it is important to respect this presentation and to understand both its development and its effectiveness; it is the self-image a person identifies with in the present. As the person learns more about her whole personality she may wish to adjust the persona to better reflect who she actually is.

I remember a very young-looking woman who came to see me with various physical symptoms as well as an underlying wish to develop herself. Her clothes were those of a teenager. She spoke in a girl's soft high voice. She came across as an innocent, cute girl just out of high school. I was amazed to learn, however, that she was in fact 30 years old, had finished university education and had already lived through many horrendous experiences in her life. As she explored herself and her life history she eventually developed a persona that was more congruent with her actual values, abilities and goals, and which was more effective in her relationships and work.

As we work directly in the body the personal history and actual personality structure will emerge naturally. The release of body armor in muscles and tissues helps to reveal the layers and patterns of the personality which can then be processed and understood in consciousness. This work is the first step toward gaining a free body, and a personality liberated from personal history.

The knowledge and practice of releasing rigid patterns of body armoring originated with the need to free malfunctioning parts of the organism, just as we instinctively rub tight shoulders to ease tension. Reich discovered that these rigid patterns in the body related directly to "character" (or personality) development. He found that the personality would open up and change as the body was freed from past stored trauma. Reich's work helped to explain the relationships between types of body armoring and corresponding "character disorders," and pointed the way toward integrative work.

Bodywork which focuses only on observable muscular and tissue rigidity or disorders, however, and does not process the material which comes off the body, can sometimes be dangerous.

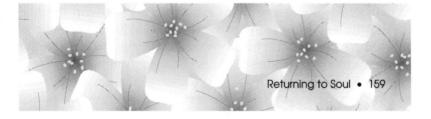

If the personality is not yet adequately understood and the ego structure is not strong enough to handle shocking information, the experience of old traumas resurfacing in the present can be intensely stressful. It could provoke personality disorientation and/or a flood of unconscious material which the person may not yet be able to accept, understand or integrate.

> *It is dangerous to restructure people simply because the restructuring goes along with a physical ideal or some theory of health. The term "normal" cannot be generalized. Each individual has his or her own norm. Process is a matter of what the Chinese call Tao. Timing a change in the body is not up to the therapist, but rather up to the person's body indications.* (Mindell, *River's Way*, 1985)

For example, if the zealous bodyworker pushes or forces through personality defenses prematurely, to expose the deep structure of the metaprogram, the resulting shock and anxiety may cause the client's body to re-armor and re-defend at this deeper level. Further, if personality patterns, habitual perspectives and attitudes toward life are not changed to keep up with the body's changes during bodywork, the body can re-establish its old patterns.

The individual with a Type A personality, geared toward high achievement, may experience momentary release from physical tension through bodywork alone. But until the basic personality structure is changed, the body will revert to the same Type A patterns soon after the bodywork is finished. Purely physical work may be temporary if it is not supported by corresponding work in consciousness

Therefore I prefer releasing the body according to the person's evolving process rather than through a prescribed formula for releasing armor. There are notable exceptions to this preference of course; for some people at certain times, or with specific conditions, a short-term, intensive program to release armor can be useful. Contemporary bodywork is evolving to incorporate more psychological understanding. There are a number of present systems which include processing the mind and emotions, such as Dr. John Upledger's Somato-Emotional release techniques and Process Acupressure. (Upledger, *Somato-Emotional Release,* 1990; Raheem, *Process Acupressure,* 1990)

Personal history—the material of the personality—can be gradually unraveled and released in the body, brought to consciousness and processed as the personality work progresses. A person comes to experience directly and exactly how the natural body and feeling responses to life were often denied or repressed to accommodate the authorities or significant others in the environment. As consciousness is brought into such buried spaces, a person begins to reclaim the truth which arises out of his own body, mind and emotions, and learns to trust that truth in the present. He can begin to understand outdated patterns of conditioning in thinking and feeling, and self-defeating behaviors which obstruct growth. As confidence in his own perceptions strengthens, consciousness will clarify. Trust for inner truth begins to replace trusting the outside. The ego can continue to develop on the solid foundation of personal, current experience. New insights and strengths gained through his explorations are anchored into the body through the bodywork, to assure integration and permanence. Gradually he learns how to assume responsibility for changing them.

DISCOVERING AND OWNING ALL PARTS OF THE PERSONALITY

During the course of personality investigation many parts within the overall personality structure will emerge. Understanding how these parts affect our lives has been extensively studied by Stone, Bandler and Grinder, Mindell and Assagioli, who termed them "subpersonalities." Some of these parts help us; they assist competence and growth. Others seem to work against us, especially those "shadow" parts that have been "disowned," that is, cut off from awareness and buried in the unconscious, from where they exert untoward effects. Some parts are destructive or simply useless, principally because they originated in stages of development which we have now outgrown.

By identifying, getting to know and consciously reowning parts of ourselves that have been disowned, we can reclaim all the energy and consciousness that were invested in them. Through conscious understanding, shadow parts that were unconscious and destructive can actually be transformed into useful allies. There are excellent techniques for identifying and integrating these parts within various psychological systems, such as Psychosynthesis (Assagioli, 1965), Neurolinguistic Programming (Bandler and Grinder, 1981), Voice Dialogue (Stone, 1978) and Process Oriented Psychology (Mindell, 1986). Since parts are frequently associated with specific body locations or symptoms, bodywork can be very helpful in releasing their energies. As "disowned" parts or subpersonalities are reoccupied, and their patterns made conscious, they can serve the wholistic purposes of a person more fully

WORK WITHIN THE DEEP STRUCTURE OF THE PERSONALITY: FREEING THE INNER CHILD

As we learned in Chapter Three, the deep structure of the personality—the metaprogram and core—was formed in childhood and holds the most fundamental influences of the entire personality. These influences affect the adult from the inner child. They are especially powerful because they are primarily unconscious and not accessible by ordinary means.

The metaprogram contains conditioning and traumas from early childhood and forms the basic foundations of the personality. The core holds imprints from the prenatal period, birth, and infancy. Together they make up the basic conditioned structure of the inner child's personality. Root traumas—the principal building blocks of neurosis—are anchored here.

Inner child work within the metaprogram and core is extremely meaningful, and a necessary part of the individuation process. In fact, these are the most powerful levels in which to effect change. Release, healing and alteration within the inner child automatically affect the whole of the personality.

This stage of exploring back into childhood, and even infancy, requires vulnerability and a kind of regression into childlike states. Generally it is best accomplished with a guide or therapist. The process can be quite frightening to the adult who has grown used to playing tough, enduring pain and defending himself through numbness. And it can be dangerous to enter this realm prematurely. A person needs enough ego strength to deal with the primal unconscious material that emerges and a bodymind that is relatively consciously connected with its own process. Defense structures, arising as "resistance," should be respected because they will usually discourage or prevent inappropriate intervention.

At the Institute for Transpersonal Psychology, where the students were deeply committed to their own personal development while training to be therapists, inner child work was essential. While there, as both student and faculty member, I observed and experienced many transformative processes that awakened the inner child. I could always tell when a student was reaching authenticity by the vulnerable and defenseless characteristics that emerged. In fact, as students advanced in the program year by year they correspondingly became more like children in certain ways—more open, loving, spontaneous and honest.

Memories of long-buried traumas from early childhood, birth, or even the prenatal period, can be revealed through sensitive body, breath, and altered state work. The destructive personality patterns, formed out of these traumas, can create a victim consciousness and a "victim body," as described by Arnold Mindell. Such patterns, imbedded into the body and the deep structure of the personality, tend to keep a person in a victim position for life, where things just "happen" to him, beyond his control. These patterns can also create a limiting "dream field" around the person as well, because they can broadcast from the deep structure of the personality right out into the energetic field around him. The dream field then attracts to the person the very situations and types of people who "victimized" him in early years. For example, the adult who was abused as a child will tend to attract abusing relationships again and again until the victim body and consciousness are cleared.

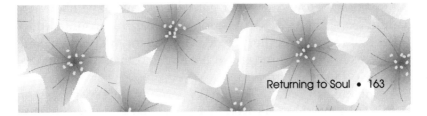

I believe that the inner child's consciousness, recorded in the body, can be most effectively regained through bodywork. In my experience, destructive personality patterns within these levels are more quickly identified, discharged and dislodged through bodywork than through verbal analysis. It has been amply demonstrated through the last decades of "talk therapy" that insight alone will not necessarily free a person from the feelings, behaviors and ideas that trip him up. Further, deep personality structure is buried in the unconscious and not accessible to ordinary awareness or analysis. Even if an analyst sees and points out (diagnosis) destructive patterns, the client will not usually be able to understand or change them because they must be altered within the unconscious and the bodymind where they occurred in the first place. Actual change in the nervous system is needed to institute new growth-promoting patterns.

As body armor softens a person can allow awareness to come closer to the inner child's original perceptions, hurts and fears. Once the numbness of armor has been penetrated, the pain of original traumas will surface. Re-experiencing such pain, is difficult but it is also the way through to freedom. Catharsis is healing and liberating when it is allowed, and even encouraged, to go all the way—that is, for the original experience to be known, felt, processed and completed. However, catharsis alone is not enough, especially if the same painful experience is repeatedly expressed, as we have seen in so many growth workshops. Such practice only imprints pain deeper into the nervous system. Once a trauma is encountered, it is best to complete the whole work of catharsis, comprehension and release of bodymind charge. If the experience is only timidly approached, or opened up in the body but not finished in consciousness, it can accumulate more energetic charge, and more armor will develop as the experience closes over again. In such a case, victim consciousness is only perpetuated. A person might consciously or unconsciously take the position, "How can I ever get well when I have had such painful experience?" That position, sometimes encountered in "over therapized" people, provides excuse for malfunction and reinforces limitations instead of healing and liberating the person toward forward growth.

Remembering and re-experiencing traumatic experiences of childhood should be followed by healing and empowerment of the natural child. We want to actually rescue the hurt child from the effects of her painful ordeals. Then we need to teach her how to reclaim her own sensibilities, speak for herself and defend herself in appropriate ways. One of the most important gains from good bodywork is the rediscovery of one's own natural responses to life, and the ability to follow the body's wisdom.

The vulnerable child phase will quite naturally pass through a dependency stage (to therapist, mate or friend), but then the process of growing up to one's own autonomy should and can be facilitated rather rapidly. The inner child needs confidence and empowerment within herself, not extended dependency. Once I met a young woman who had been reparented by a psychologist, who was certainly a better parent than the abusive and neglecting originals. In this case the woman had now become completely dependent on the psychologist, however, and wasn't learning to trust her own needs and sensibilities.

REBIRTHING, REPARENTING AND REPATTERNING

Healing and/or restructuring of old traumatic patterns should accompany or follow the opening and releasing of energy held within them. This phase is sometimes neglected in therapies that mainly emphasize catharsis or just "getting it out." Simply discovering and expressing old wounds can harmfully restimulate their pain and the accompanying messages in the body if they are not resolved and restructured within a new understanding. In fact, I tell my students not to enter a severe trauma within the body unless they can shepherd it all the way through to resolution. Wounds and limiting patterns should be transformed into valuable resources, otherwise their expression can become an excuse for neurotic endurance. For example, we want to avoid reinforcing the feelings and behaviors of the abused child who can blame the negative mother endlessly for not getting on with life in the present. As the deep personality is healed and restructured, the victim body and the bindings of personal history can be liberated. A positive mother force can be built from nurturing models, from the past or in the present, and the person's own internal mother resources. A client who had been learning how to take care of her inner child said to me, "Now I know how to mother myself." Negative mother messages and influences will gradually be diluted within a stream of nurturing support.

Bodywork is usually essential during such depth transformation processes, to release metaprogram traumas from the tissues, and to assist in restructuring them in the consciousness. Adult and/or soul consciousness is used to communicate with the helpless child, and to bring it those qualities—such as love, protection, strength or support—that were originally missing in childhood. There is a profoundly loving Indian guru who does her world service by traveling around and simply holding people in her heart love.

Depth transformation can be accomplished by bringing new perspectives and/or creating new realities around the traumas. This is accomplished through various depth techniques, such as reparenting, reprogramming, healing-of-memories, visualization, prayer, rebirthing, affirmations and intention. In my experience these techniques are most effective when they are done with the client in an altered state, at the level of the unconscious where the trauma occurred in the first place, and with loving support from the consciousness of both therapist and client.

Baby therapy is often required to make up for the open-hearted mother love that many babies missed. There may not be a direct replacement for the body-imprinted safety , love and bliss that a baby feels at her mother's breast. But it is possible to deliver a healthy substitute for that experience through healing work in the body, or baby-focused self-attention. When clients are working with their inner babies I often ask them to imagine holding their inner baby at night when they go to bed. They do this for several weeks, until a new impression in the baby's body can take hold.

After strong reprogramming work within her inner child, a client who had a very neglectful mother had a dream in which she was a baby. The baby said "no more cold milk." This dream signaled to me that the adult mother within the client was now taking over the job of nurturing her inner child.

A psychologically sophisticated client who was struggling with her inner baby's lack of mother love and contact, asked me to do an experimental session of holding her. Both of us were edgy about doing the session and about its possible effects. But we took the risk. I held her for five hours, almost completely in silence, before she had enough. We were amazed at how deeply it helped her sense of body safety, belonging and self-esteem. She never required another session like that, and I learned a great deal about the value of concentrated attention delivered to the body.

Once a client and I discovered an ingenious way to bring safety and comfort to her baby body. While exploring her infancy, we found that she frequently left her body to avoid the feelings of neglect and pain she felt within it. Through our work she was now willing, as an adult, to completely re-occupy that baby body, but somehow the boundaries of it had been lost to her consciousness. She asked me if I could press her back into the body. So I began pressing my hands into her body, somewhat like I used to squeeze my own babies. I started at her feet and squeezed through the whole body, ending at the head. She breathed a great sigh of relief as I finished and said, "Oh, that's better. Now I'm fully in here."

Through such means, a traumatic birth, prenatal wounding or early childhood traumas can be literally transformed within the body. I have directed and participated in many rebirths in which the original painful and frightening experience was transformed into a welcoming beginning to life. Until very recently it was quite uncommon for a baby to be ushered into life by a welcoming committee, including loving, accepting parents and a nurturing medical team. It was more usual for the mother to be "gone" on anesthetic, the father to be nowhere near the scene and the doctor to be too busy with the mechanics of an unconscious birth to also deliver loving reception.

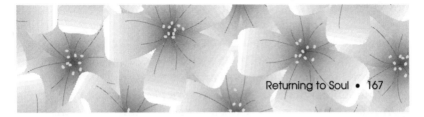

I remember one rebirth which completely changed a man's subsequent life. His original birth was long, hard and painful. At the end, when the mother discovered he was a boy instead of the girl she wanted, she ordered the nurses to "take him away" Needless to say he felt a lifelong shame, about hurting his mother and about not being acceptable. The rebirth was fortunately done in a group so that there was a strong loving energy and a number of players to re-do the experience. Everyone spontaneously offered some special gift to him as he was re-birthing. One woman called out, "Oh, it's a boy! Isn't that wonderful!" Another said "Welcome to this world. We're so glad you came." Two other women held him close to their bodies after the birth. A creative man wrote, in huge letters, "It's a boy!" on the ground outside our group room for all to see as we left. This man was quite different thereafter. He had a sense of power he had never before felt in this life. He changed his way of relating to people. He felt able to actually carry out a strong life purpose he had dreamed of but wasn't sure he could accomplish.

4. TURNING DAMAGE INTO RESOURCE

As healing and restructuring progresses in the deep structures, crippling damage can be turned into evolutionary resource. For example, Milton Erickson, the great hypnotherapist, called problems and traumas the "roughage" of life. He transformed his own early crippling experiences of color blindness, tone deafness, dyslexia, and later polio into rich resources. While still a teenager recovering from polio, he used his "handicaps" to drive his consciousness deep into the body and the mind to find out just how they worked at microlevels. Much later, after a severe struggle through medical school, he employed his very subtle learnings to assist his patients in ways that others had never considered.

In my own practice many clients have transformed metaprogram material from traumas into strengths. For example, a woman learned at a soul level that she had brought herself to abusive parents in order to turn to God very early in life. With this understanding she was able to see her painful experiences as training rather than victimization. Another woman discovered that she had chosen an early crazy and unpredictable environment so that she would experience the most base levels of human existence and develop compassion for them. Such information is very important in helping a person move from the victim position to one of self-guided mastery.

A woman told me the seemingly horrible story of her life. She was born in a mental institution to a mother and father who were inmates. The cord was wrapped around her neck when she was born. Surviving that, she shortly contracted a serious illness which kept her debilitated through much of her childhood. Of course she had no loving parenting and was shifted about from one relative's home to another. In adulthood she found herself in one abusing relationship after another until she was finally almost shattered. Near complete defeat, she sought healing and eventually turned toward a path of self-exploration and spiritual growth. I asked her incredulously, "Why did you stay in life when you could have got out so many times?" Her answer: "To experience life, the beauty of it. The sun in the trees, birds flying, sunrises." This woman had turned an impossible history, from a clinical point of view, into wisdom.

5. WORK WITHIN THE CORE OF THE BODY AND THE SELF

As metaprogram material is released from the body the vital core of the person can be exposed. The core contains that free and spontaneous bodymind state of the yet unconditioned child, the "divine child" state, which is very close to the soul. At this level all beings are unique, creative and loving, and they are connected with the Divine. Here, beneath all the traumas and dramas of personal history, is a priceless reservoir of natural and transcendent resources, derived from both individual soul wisdom and the collective unconscious of humankind through the centuries.

In the core, one is whole. Images and metaphors which arise from this realm are pre-verbal and wholistic and they reflect the very essence of the person, and of life. According to Jung:

> *They serve to produce an inner order....They express the idea of a safe refuge, of inner reconciliation and wholeness....When we*

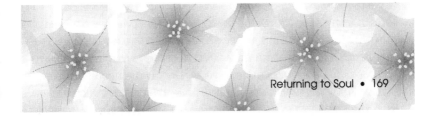

penetrate a little more deeply below the surface of the psyche, we come upon historical layers which are not just dead dust, but alive and continuously active in everyone—maybe to a degree that we cannot imagine in the present state of our knowledge.
(Jung, *The Archetypes and the Collective Unconscious*, 1959)

These images, metaphors and symbols can be powerfully affirming and healing because they are at the very foundation of consciousness from where they can affect the whole system of body, mind and emotions at once. Great creative freedom is available at this level because the mind is unfettered by conditioned patterns; thus it can be laser-focused through intention. Through this core consciousness personality patterns can be restructured and new realities created around them.

Clearing and repatterning of the deep personality structure bring much greater freedom in which the person can experience all parts of himself and express them fully. During the course of such wholistic process work, one comes to rely on the truth of one's own feelings, body sensations and thoughts. One can gain choice over more of one's life. Personal history can become an objective resource, the "prima materia" of wisdom, rather than a limiting program. A person is then able to institute new behaviors and new ways of being. He has gained the freedom, and built the strength, to follow his own soul. Such a person is now liberated from the fix of fate and can instead claim a destiny.

Every free individual lends greater possibility for global survival and reconstruction. Individuals who are liberated will not follow false teachers. They can be free of the prevalent unconscious twentieth-century conditioning toward self-destruction; instead they can pursue a conscious process toward creative growth. In his important book, *The Path of Least Resistance*, Robert Fritz described a hope for humankind, engendered through creative individuals:

*One of the most important lessons I have learned in the past
fifteen years of teaching the creative process concerns the true
nature of people. When people are united with their real power—
the power to create what they want to create—they always
choose what is highest in humanity. They choose good health,
exceptional relationships, and love, and relevant life purpose,
and peace, and challenges worthy of the human spirit. People, I
have come to discover, are profoundly good. (1984)*

6. SOUL WORK

Fortunately it is not necessary to clear all the deep structures
of the personality, or even all the obstructive patterns, before we
can engage in soul work. Rather, we have found that seeking
active soul participation will lend a perspective and much greater
expansion for the ongoing personality work. The soul dimension
prevents a person's development from being completely limited
by the bindings of the childhood and opens up the grace of
spiritual resource.

Transpersonal Integration requests soul participation from
the beginning of the work and seeks to facilitate conscious soul
contact as early as possible. I am convinced through my experience with hundreds of clients that this contact is both accessible
and desirable. Phyllis Krystal, psychotherapist and international
teacher of her soul-centered work, has found the same thing with
hundreds around the world. She says,

*I set forth a method of counselling based on the understanding
that our true identity is not, as many people believe, the temporary and imperfect body or the personality. It is much more than
that. It is the inner, permanent and perfect Self....Most people are
unaware of It because It is hidden from sight, unlike the outer
physical form.* (Krystal, *Cutting More Ties That Bind*, 1990)

Once invited in, the soul will begin to influence our process.
As soon as the client is beyond the most beginning stages, and the
"static" of the personality is somewhat sorted out and calmed
down, the still small voice of the soul can begin to reveal itself.
Soul guidance is then requested during each session. This deep
wisdom becomes an important component of the ongoing psychological work. As it is respected, the inner spiritual life is
strengthened.

Even before there is extensive personality clearing a person may be brought to the deeper truth of the soul through great shock or spiritual experience. For example, the death or loss of a loved one, serious illness, or an intense meditation experience can drive consciousness into profound levels where it will question the very roots of existence. "Why an I here?" "What is the meaning of this suffering?" "What is death?" Such experiences can open temporary doorways directly into the soul and provide important opportunities for self-realization. Sometimes just within a few hours or days, such an opening can change the course of a life. Major insights, decisions or behavior changes at that time can direct a person toward more meaning and purpose in life.

A number of clients have demonstrated that it is possible to rediscover the soul and access its direct guidance to actualize its purpose. Subtle soul messages show up in every day life, and certainly are evident in the normal course of psychotherapy, through dreams, hunches, unconsciously engendered artistic productions and fantasies. At first such messages are hesitant, illusive, even subliminal. They surface in fragmented bits through the dreams, waking images or memories. But when we listen to these messages, and take them seriously, they will become more frequent and clear; soon they will become an easy part of our ongoing therapy process. Vital spiritual practice is also encouraged, to feed the soul and to cultivate the stillness through which it can whisper. Soul food is not a common commodity; it must be sought after and cultivated.

Gradually soul messages will come forward more strongly into the vessel of reception provided within the therapist-client relationship. Soul communication and soul awareness can become tangible realities rather than spiritual abstraction. For example a woman reported the following experience during a time when she was beginning to do soul work:

While lying down in a meditative state I had a luminous experi-
ence of being the soul body, shining through the physical body
for a minute or so. I could feel this much larger, lighter body
extending above, beyond and through the physical body. For a
moment I realized that although I inhabit, and am, this body, I
am also much more than it.

A person can be led into direct soul contact through an altered state. I can tell when this is possible through the body's energy condition. There is a balanced, steady energy state which follows deep relaxation in the body, mind and emotions. Often there is a reverent stillness in the atmosphere. When this condition occurs, it is possible to speak directly to the soul and to ask it for information and guidance. As the person speaks from the soul, there is a quiet but firm assurance in the voice and a quality of objectivity that sounds different from ordinary speech. The person remains completely conscious, although in a deep state, and may use personal volition at any time.

At first a person may be shy and unsure of the information from this level. This is natural and important. It is necessary to test it out in daily life by applying soul guidance through taking concrete actions and discovering the results. Through repeated contact with this level the client learns how to consult the soul fairly readily; she knows the state and how to get there.

The depth of soul work sometimes leads a person into ancient themes and patterns that can't be traced to the personality of the present. Mythic images, teachings or obstructions can crop up as "ancestral" imprints that affect the person. I have met the "sin" of Eve theme in many women's depth processes, even though the contemporary woman may have no intellectual affinity for that "original sin" idea. Through the Subud *latihan*, people have experienced the "purification" of their ancestors within their individual spiritual practice. And I have encountered the influence of powerful ancestors, sometimes several generations removed, within the work of a number of clients. Investigation of "past lives" may be useful, either to clear obstructive soul patterns from the past, or to recover valuable talents and skills from the past to use in the present life. I do past life work within the context of the ongoing therapy when such experiences naturally arise. Whether this kind of material comes from actual past lives, in a linear evolutionary pattern, or from mythic impressions out of the collective unconscious, is not yet known. But these experiences do occur and they provide consciousness with symbolic meanings which help delineate growth steps. When these past life experiences occur, it is important to respect the material and to clear or heal whatever obstruction there is within it. After a person has experienced several past lives, and often the very explicit deaths that have ended them, he usually gains a serene sense of the eternity of life, and the temporality of death.

Sometimes it is possible to elicit soul purpose as we work at core levels. Usually clients have an inkling when they are ready to receive this information. We may discuss the possibility at a conscious level and then ask for the life's purpose while in an altered state. Examples of purposes that have been reported by clients are: "I came this time to heal the relationships with my father and younger sister (both known to the client in a past life) and to learn forgiveness"; "I am here to practice healing as a service to humanity and to heal myself through this service"; "My purpose is to bring forth those psychic abilities I had long ago in the service of humanity and to learn not to misuse them as I did before."

Gradually the focus of motivation within a person is shifted from personality to soul. Adaptation to outer achievement, approval and control become less compelling and one develops a deep need to be true to the Self.

Spiritual Development

As the individuating person becomes more soul-centered than personality-driven, spiritual and psychological work begin to merge. Outer work on the personality can continue to open pathways into the core, and inner spiritual work becomes more important.

One will naturally be drawn toward transpersonal questions—"Why am I here?" "How am I related to the whole of life?" "What is the right way of living for me?" "What is my relationship to God and how do I cultivate it?" The need for spiritual direction will be felt. Spiritual practice, suited to the individual nature, should be encouraged at this time. It can contribute enormously to the process because soul guidance will emerge more clearly through transpersonal attunement. The higher chakras are activated by spiritual practice and their awakening will bring greater strength and clarity to assist soul realization. Spiritual practice facilitates working from the inside out, while psychological work proceeds from the outside in. As the two combine in a transpersonal approach, the whole person is revealed more fully.

Spiritual practice can also bring an influx of spiritual energy, known as the "infilling of the Holy Spirit" in Christian terms. This higher vibration energy is very powerful. It can effect miraculous healing—in body, emotions, mind or spirit. It can also provoke a "purification" process, or "healing crisis," in which old negative material that obstructs the soul is flushed up into body and consciousness and needs to be worked through and released. Purification can take place in dramatic and often frightening episodes, or it can extend over a longer, smoother period. But unlike useless suffering, it bears the fruits of soul realization and spiritual consciousness over time.

As spiritual energy is integrated into spiritual consciousness a person can begin to receive inspirations—explanations and instructions—or "callings" to tasks that go beyond the personal. "Miracles"—events that have no logical or even plausible explanation—can happen. It is possible to "practice the presence of God," that is, to exist in a state of inspired rapture in which one feels, hears or sees the evidence of God in all things.

Many mystics through the ages have reported such states of being. But most often they have found it necessary to separate themselves from the ordinary world in order to maintain them. They have provided examples for humankind from a distance, through writing (which is always inadequate, as they admit, since such consciousness states cannot be actually described in words), or stories told by their followers.

Yet it is possible to actualize the fruits of spiritual energy and guidance in ordinary life. After all, daily practice within the life one has is the true ground of spiritual development. And in adverse conditions spiritual resources provide the most fundamental solace and strength. I encountered an amazing example of the transformation of suffering into spiritual gold at the First International Holistic Health Conference in India. There I had the great privilege of meeting Dr. Chodyrak, who was the physician of the Dalai Lama in Tibet before the Chinese invasion. He was captured by the Chinese before he could leave Tibet. For 22 years he was not only held captive but tortured unmercifully. During all that time he held fast to his inner spiritual practice as a way of coping with impossible conditions. He meditated and used inner rituals to withstand torture, without harboring bitterness. Rather, he said that he could only feel compassion for his torturers since he knew what karma they were engendering. He practiced medicine for fellow prisoners as well as for the guards. Finally he was released to join the Dalai Lama in India. He was one of the most humble, radiant and compassionate men I have ever met. His ordeals had taken him to a very deep wisdom, strength and healing ability.

When a person is able to align with the soul and to actualize spiritual practice through an activated system of body, mind and emotions, he is truly whole. As all parts are enlivened, the soul can illuminate them from within. The awakened and free body has the power and flexibility to carry out the soul's destiny. Finally the personality is willing to follow soul.

Individuation Leads to Wholeness

Awakening in body, mind, emotions and soul brings a person to wholeness. Awareness, vitality and volition in all these parts enable one to respond to life from the complete and whole human system that one is, rather than from the fragmented perspective one has learned through conditioning. As the integrity and needs of each part are accepted, a person can responsibly create his own wellness and growth.

Individuation then becomes a continuous process of reclaiming the truth and power from all parts of the being and learning how to radiate soul illumination out from the soul center through them. Freedom is at hand; a person can "get out from under" the tent of conditioning and soar into his own individuality as a liberated being, who can follow his own truth.

Wholeness leads to a remarkable kind of consciousness which is "enlightened" (having aliveness and light) in all parts. A person experiences the capacity to radiate soul energy, or light, fully and freely through the cells of the physical body, the activated neurons of the mind, and through the waves of emotion. Out of the authentic experience of his own complete system, one is able to wholistically perceive What Is. Theories of reality are replaced by direct knowing, about oneself and the environment. In *River's Way*, Arnold Mindell described such an individual:

> *What will happen to the individual when his ability to perceive increases? If experience is an indicator, increasing ability at picking up signals and courage in working with their implications will liberate the individual from false teachers and healers. Neither knowledge, luck nor intelligence, but expanded sensitivity to the wisdom of one's own process creates the independence of a congruent personality. (1985)*

Through knowing himself directly, wholistically, a person gains the capacity to respond to the ever-changing truth of the moment, without translation through learned behavior. Lao Tzu (in the Ni Hua-Ching translation) described such consciousness:

> *To be is to be true. The muchness and suchness of truth is included in this very second. If you miss the truth of this moment, a thousand galloping horses cannot catch up with it. The totality of truth presents itself to you every time you blink your eyes. It can dance on the tip of your eyelash. It is as far as the eyes can see and as much as the mind can hold. It exists in every moment of time and every bit of space. (Tao Te Ching, 1985)*

So it is that the person who is awake to all of himself can be fully alert in the moment, perceive the whole truth of it, and respond with maximum efficient action. He can flow with the Tao.

A client who was well into her individuation process and in contact with her feelings, mind and soul recorded the following session which exemplifies whole being consciousness:

During this session I was working to integrate my inner and outer life, so that the energy inside me can be expressed congruently through my physical form. I had been experiencing some armoring, tightness and rigidity, in my outer musculature. It seemed like a block to the aliveness I am feeling deep inside.

During the session images of sixteen paintings I have just finished drift across the screen of my mind. Three float above the other thirteen, displaying an extra brightness, or luminosity. The three luminous pieces are: Warrior, Phoenix and Isis.

These three paintings fascinate me. I see that they came about through no conscious planning, in their own time. I see that the other pieces had to be painted to prepare the way for the more luminous ones. The psyche has to work on more superficial issues before the pathway can be cleared for deeper messages to come through. I see that these three paintings were all born out of an intense chaotic energy: Warrior began with agitation and anger; Phoenix emerged out of physical pain and a dark dream; Isis appeared after a psychological descent into the realm of the Dark Goddess.

As my body's energy is being balanced, Warrior stops floating outside my body and anchors itself in my pelvic girdle. There the image pulsates, the vibrancy of the colors translating into waves of energy that enliven my first three chakras. I feel an inner yang strength that goes far beyond what the outer image of the male Indian conveys to my mind.

I then sense Isis in my head, energizing my throat, brow and crown chakras. The powerful goddess informs my body of her ancient wisdom and I experience a profound spiritual harmony. Phoenix next lights in my heart, and a sense of wholeness envelopes me. My heart chakra becomes the vital link between my lower and higher centers. As I embody these powerful archetypes in my body, I appreciate all of the creative forces I have "unleashed" in my paintings. I am redeeming the energy of my creativity, bringing back into my body that which I had previously projected onto my canvasses, redeeming the power and the force that created the images in the first place.

This redemption process fills me with a deep reverence for my spiritual practice, which opens the channel between myself and the universe. When the energy is caught in the unconscious, I am physically asleep. When it is projected onto objects or beings outside myself, I am only half awake. My spiritual practice, whether in the form of meditation or painting, is the vehicle with which I become one with the Tao, or the flow in and out. It allows me to manifest my Essence and to give me the experience of Presence, the ultimate pulse of Spirit.

The Great Tao Within and Beyond the Self

One who knows the soul will also know the Great Spirit, or the Tao—that vitalizing, benevolent wave of the universe which interpenetrates All That Is, including the individual soul. Personal wholeness brings a feeling of unity with that Spirit. A sense of separateness—from oneself, others and the environment—is replaced by an inner attunement to a great Natural Order. Surrender to that order—the final stage of all spiritual practice—becomes possible and appealing. A sense of well-being and integrity will automatically accompany this stage.

In the late twentieth century, when our very planetary existence hangs in the balance, we must cultivate such spiritual consciousness within, to link us harmonically to the Universal Order. Now, we must claim the ancient promise from Jeremiah:

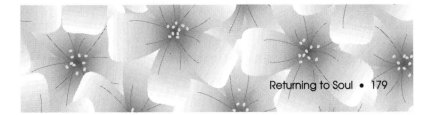

"I will put my law in their inward parts, and write it in their hearts....for they shall all know Me." We need practical mystics in our time (Mother Teresa is a notable example) who can bring spiritual guidance into concrete reality.

In addition to awakening higher states of consciousness to tap the universal guidance that is available to us, we must also be able to integrate these states and their directions through the body, mind and emotions and out into the world in concrete ways. Hence the psychological foundation of the spiritual work is essential. The influx of higher energy through an imbalanced or unprepared personality can cause an even greater personality disorder. Such a recipient may become, at best, simply an ineffectual dreamer.

It is important here to emphasize that this stage of self-actualization and transpersonal development is little known in ordinary life on this planet. It is not yet a collective phenomenon. We are attempting to describe a quality of awareness and living that seems to be the next evolutionary step for humankind. Models are scarce, it generally takes a wide search of spiritual biographies to find them. Yet there are many among the "Aquarian conspiracy" who are seeking, and finding, ways to define and live this higher level of human development. It requires taking risks, venturing into unfamiliar territories. It brings a massive shift in perspective which must be accommodated by new ways of being with oneself and the world. For example, great energy intensity, the sometimes searing awareness of facing the unveiled truth, the insecurity of following one's own truth and the loneliness of standing apart from the collective—these aspects and more accompany the journey of being true to the soul and the Great Tao.

In *Memories, Dreams and Reflections* (1961), Carl Jung described how it was for him to follow God through his own truth:

Nobody could rob me of the conviction that it was enjoined upon me to do what God wanted and not what I wanted. That gave me the strength to go my own way. Often I had the feeling that in all decisive matters I was no longer among men, but was alone with God.

The individual soul, as a part of the living Spirit, can create through inspiration from the Spirit. Inner attunement with the living Spirit, through prayer and meditation, can bring creative ideas and solutions to problems that go beyond the ordinary mind. As the individual soul aligns more and more with universal Spirit, a person can become an instrument of universal purpose. Co-creation with Spirit—always original, fresh, and new in the moment—becomes possible. And in this way one's own purpose can serve the whole.

Great spiritual projects, movements and services are inspired through the receptivity of one or a few individuals who are available to Spirit. Remember the global impact of such single individuals as Martin Luther King, Jr.; Anwar Sadat; and His Holiness, the Dalai Lama. My own teacher, Mohammad Subuh, spread an enormously valuable spiritual resource out into the world by following his destiny to bring the spiritual practice of Subud to thousands. Less recognized but just as important are the contributions that millions of spiritual servants—ordinary good people—make to the betterment of humankind through their daily life services. In fact, service and co-creation with Spirit probably offer the greatest hope in today's world for solving our seemingly insoluble planetary problems.

In *River's Way*, (1985) Arnold Mindell writes about the implications of being the "total self," as it aligns with the great creative Order, or the Tao:

Now Tao is an experience. It is your ally, an inner certainty related to the overall state of the world which detaches you from the opinions of your group. Talmudic literature, American Indian tradition and Taoist stories remind you of the powerful and ameliorating effect of this ally. They predict that if one person gets himself together while being in this real world, that the whole world will fall into order.

Summary

The return to soul is an extra-ordinary journey that involves nothing less than the whole person's commitment to his full development. It will take the seeker beyond stages of fulfilling collective values and achieving worldly success into the unique path of his own individuality, and the process of individuation.

In this chapter psycho-spiritual development was explored. It was shown that progressive growth goes through stages of individuation, in which a person learns to follow his own nature toward greater wholeness and eventual self realization. Therapeutic methods for facilitating that growth were explained in general and within the context of Transpersonal Integration.

The stage of psychological/personality work was related to uncovering and releasing the layers of personal history within the body—from the most recent experiences back to the very beginning of life and the core of the body. It was shown that the realization of the whole self occurs through the awakening of all parts.

Spiritual development was defined as an awakening of the individual soul, in which a person becomes soul-centered and soul-directed in the process of realization of individual destiny. Free, spiritually-directed individuals are proposed as possibly the greatest hope for a humankind that is stumbling beneath the self-destructive behaviors of centuries. For it is only through a higher human development, connected to and guided by Spirit, that we can gain the life-preserving and love-enhancing attitudes and practices that will lead our species into its next evolutionary step.

CHAPTER SEVEN

TRANSPERSONAL INTEGRATION AND ITS IMPLICATIONS FOR THE TRANSPERSONAL THERAPIST

Transpersonal Integration is designed to assist with the unfolding of the whole person and to harmonize the personality with the inner guidance of the soul. It requires the knowledge and skill to work adeptly in body, mind, emotions and soul and to follow them simultaneously according to the individual, wholistic process. Thus the Transpersonal Integration therapist needs firm grounding in physical, psychological and spiritual work.

I believe Transpersonal Integration can also offer useful guidelines for transpersonal psychotherapy which can be translated into the various modalities used within the field.

In *Beyond Ego: Transpersonal Dimensions in Psychology*, (1980) Vaughan and Walsh describe certain desirable qualities for the transpersonal therapist as follows:

1) modeling by the therapist for the client, which is closely linked to Karma yoga, the yoga of service;
2) work by the therapist on his own consciousness;
3) a relationship-building attitude, rather than the traditional impersonal doctor-patient role.

They conclude by saying:

Working with one's own consciousness (that of the therapist) becomes a primary responsibility, for the growth of one participant is seen as facilitating that of the other....In Transpersonal therapy, the values and attitudes of the therapist are thus of crucial importance, and the effects of modeling can be recognized not only in overt behavior but in subtle attitudes as well....Because we are both the tools and the models for what we have to offer, it is imperative that we seek to live and be that which we would offer our clients.

Within the context of Transpersonal Integration I wish to draw some additional guidelines that could be helpful for transpersonal psychotherapists. These are described below within the realms of relationship, energy, body, spiritual and wholistic awareness.

Relationship Awareness

The relationship between therapist and client is a living, interactive process that develops its own character and resources during the work. As Vaughan and Walsh have recommended, a relationship-building attitude is preferred to the traditional doctor/patient mode. Relationship skills often need to be developed, particularly when the therapist has been trained within the traditional model, where the therapist is the authority, or at least "helper," with all the answers, and the client is in some sense the "underdog." In actual fact, the client has all the answers about her own process, even though the therapist may need to teach her how to access them.

In Process Work, Arnold Mindell has delineated a whole spectrum of attitudes and skills for relationship work which are quite different from traditional psychotherapy. The Process

Worker is required to master these skills and I cannot recommend them highly enough, for any helper. For example, the Process Worker sees the work between client and therapist as a team effort in which both are constantly learning. He pays careful and specific attention to feedback from the client, respects it completely and integrates it, in the moment, into the process. He brings his own feelings, thoughts and experiences into the process when they seem meaningful. He processes any discomfort, tangle or confusion between them at the time it occurs.

The therapist who brings such refined relationship awareness and skills into the work can foster a developing climate of trust. Deep work, within the metaprogram and core of the personality, or in spiritual development, can only be done within a vessel of profound trust. As they test and trust each other, therapist and client can build an intimacy, and a commitment to truth, that can support truly transformative work.

Energy Awareness

Awareness of the client's energy will assist the therapist's attunement.

It has been shown how the meridian and chakra energy systems of the body interpenetrate all realms of the whole being and how they reflect states of consciousness. While the material of the body is reasonably static, energy moves and emanates through it. In fact, the entire person, from the soul center out through the personality, is constantly broadcasting its patterns out through the energy field. An adept who can read the field directly will know a great deal about the person's personality structure and soul vibration. This field can be felt by the therapist, either directly, through hand passes, or simply in the atmosphere. In fact, it is a demonstrated experience in Process Work that the therapist can be temporarily overwhelmed by the client's field—

he may think or feel things that come from the client and not himself. The client's general energy field will indicate vitality, or lack of it, and the level of his committed presence. Paying attention to the energy from the client's body, especially to the seven chakras along the midline, can give the therapist an immediate impression of where process is moving or obstructed. Generally, the session will be most productive if static energy can be released and moved. This does not necessarily require direct bodywork. Addressing the issues related to the obstructed chakra area can often promote movement.

Therapy can be greatly facilitated through explicit energy work within the client's body if the therapist observes noticeable imbalances within the body or emotions, as described in this book. Examples of effective energy modalities are: acupuncture, acupressure, chakra energy balancing and Zero Balancing. The client can also be taught simple touch and meditative techniques to facilitate energy balance.

The therapist's energy system directly affects the state of the client. When two people interact in close proximity, as in psychotherapy, their energies intermingle. The "modeling" by therapist for client, which Vaughan and Walsh refer to, has concrete meaning in terms of energy. If the therapist's energy systems are reasonably balanced and strong they will have a health-supporting effect on the client. But if they are seriously imbalanced or weak, the session can be diminished.

Bodyworkers are usually aware that the state of their own body health, strength and energy has a direct bearing on the quality of their work. Acupuncturists are taught that they should not treat clients if they are ill or seriously imbalanced. Body touching, of course, brings the bodyworker into deeper contact with a client than does talking with him. Nevertheless, it is important for the psychotherapist to know that he is constantly emanating who and where he is through his energy system and field. By building and harmonizing his own energy, the therapist will automatically assist his clients more completely.

The energy factor gives specific meaning to the quality of "presence," so important in therapy. Through his presence, which is strongly a function of energy, the therapist can influence his client toward balance and harmony, or toward less desirable states. Further, the presence of the therapist radiates and "collects" in his consulting room, which can build an environmental vessel for health. Many healers carefully create an empowering and healing environment.

Two experiences of the healing environment come to mind.

When I walk into Dr. Fritz Smith's office there is a feeling of peace and healing. As I wait for an appointment I watch his secretary and nurse. They are light, cheerful and loving, even though they are busy. It is delightful to be near them. We exchange pleasantries. We laugh. I watch old people who are not feeling well enter the office. As they sit, they seem to relax into a more comfortable state. When they leave the office they look calmer and stronger. When Dr. Smith greets them and me, he smiles. There is a sparkle in his eyes. I feel better immediately when I see him and feel his presence.

I consulted Master Ni, Hua Ching. In the heart of Los Angeles, his office was serene. There was a sense of stillness and lightness within his rooms even though the clamor of the city was just outside the door. When Master Ni came in, I was startled by the youth and lightness in his face. He moved swiftly, deftly. His presence was like a gentle breeze. He placed several needles deep into my shoulder. The needles hurt and energy rushed through my body. But I felt calmed and uplifted. Master Ni laughed several times during my short stay. His laughter was like a balm. As he removed the needles he patted my shoulder ever so lightly and said, "Now you take care of yourself, okay You will be all right." And I immediately knew that I would be.

Body Awareness

Work in consciousness requires body awareness and body release.

As we have seen, the conditioned patterns that are obstructive to transpersonal growth and self-actualization are lodged in the body. It would be valuable for the transpersonal psycho-therapist to know something about how obstructed, and released, bodies look and move. Minimally, the therapist can learn to "read" the parts of the body and their likely psychological association. During work with a client, it is very useful to notice the constant reflections in the body of the psychological process.

Although it is not necessary for transpersonal psychothera-pists to be bodyworkers, some understanding of body armoring, the types of material stored in parts of the body and psycho-physical patterns can be extremely helpful in assisting the client's whole growth process. Sometimes it may be necessary to refer the client to bodywork, particularly when psychological disor-ders result from fixed armoring in the body. It is unlikely that such disorders will dissolve through talk therapy alone.

In addition to the freeing function of bodywork it can also greatly help consolidate new learning. It has been my experience that an insight or new behavior is truly "owned" and made permanent when it is anchored into the body. That is, when a person is able to feel a new learning in the body, and act it out from the body, then the learning is securely imprinted into behavior.

It is entirely possible for a client to be lodged in emotional or mental fixations that are primarily caused by a weakened or diseased body. The therapist needs to be able to either give appropriate information about caring for the body, or refer the client to an appropriate health professional. The therapist can also advise her client about the interrelationships of body, mind, emotions and soul. This wholistic counseling will help preclude unnecessary physical and psychological pain, and hasten re-covery.

The therapist needs to care for his own body. The therapist who is aware of his own body will have greater sensitivity to the physical condition of his client. Bodywork can be extremely informative, as well as healthy and freeing, for the professional helper. The therapist who has released armored patterns within his own body will be more easily aware of similar patterns in clients' bodies. And his own freed body will model vitality and physical liberation for the client. Conversely, the unreleased body of the therapist harbors distorted energy patterns which encourage projection onto the client.

Spiritual Awareness

Traditional psychology works with mental, emotional, and sometimes physical problems to adjust dysfunction and promote growth in any or all of these realms. Consequently, there are many good psychologists who do not address the soul level, and this is appropriate. Many life problems can be solved by new and truthful information, clear thinking and a sympathetic ear. When a person enters a transpersonal state of development, however, and wishes to find her own soul, she may need a therapist with spiritual awareness and knowledge to guide her journey for awhile. Or, the person who experiences a spiritual emergence, or "crisis," that can look like a psychotic episode may seek a transpersonal therapist who is familiar with spiritual developments. In the last few years the Spiritual Emergence Network has drawn attention to the fact that many people have been inappropriately put on medication or even placed in mental institutions when they were actually experiencing the disorientation that sometimes accompanies spiritual awakening. In these times, when spiritual development is so greatly needed, spiritual work and soul attunement are necessary.

The first task for the transpersonal therapist who wishes to work at a soul level is to align himself with his own soul strength and purpose. Work on himself, through spiritual attunement and practice, is essential. Vitality of Spirit requires nourishment at a soul level. The liberation of his own soul will help the therapist to bring the wisdom and vitality of living Spirit to his client. The awakened soul radiates a vital presence, out through the body and into the field around him, which stirs other souls. An alive soul is also more sensitive to soul signals from others.

Communication with the client's soul, and the discovery of its purpose, can be facilitated directly by the transpersonal therapist. It is a gradual, delicate and fruitful process. I have discovered certain therapist attitudes and techniques which assist this process:

The therapist will need to recognize the sovereignty of the client's soul. This will include an absolute respect for the individuality, and the Divinity, of the client's soul, as well as his own.

The therapist will need to recognize and have knowledge about the different stages of soul expression. Souls are of different ages and purposes which have corresponding growth needs. For example, it may be necessary and appropriate for one soul to be completely involved in a religious life, including extensive dogma, ritual and church commitment, whereas another soul may need to be divorced from religious life. A soul's life task may be global (as with Gandhi) or it may be specifically personal. The therapist will realize that all soul purposes are equally sacred and he will find the ways to facilitate the particular purpose(s) of his client.

The childhood dream—one which stands out dramatically in memory—can give valuable clues to the "myth" or life purpose of the individual. First identified by Jung, and recently pursued in research by Arnold Mindell, this kingpin experience is an indelible, very early dream which might have occurred only once, with great impact, or recurred many times. It can be identified by the insistent nature of its images, its haunting tone, its emotional charge or its luminous quality. Mindell has found, in working with hundreds of such dreams, that they invariably describe a theme or task that lies at the very center of a person's process, around which the life tends to orient. He has also discovered that chronic body symptoms often relate to this dream. When it can be worked with consciously it can shed light on soul purpose.

Certain "extra-ordinary" information sources, para-psychological and/or spiritual, can sometimes provide useful keys for understanding the individual soul pattern. These include the astrological horoscope, psychic readings and other oracular tools such as Tarot or I Ching consultations. The horoscope gives a birth map that shows tendencies toward talents, life tasks and limitations to be overcome for the life. Similarly, a well-trained palm reader can find life strengths and obstructions within the palm of the hand. A "good" psychic (meaning one who has true extra-sensory perception, integrity and has done his own psychological work) can read patterns within the psyche that are usually outside the client's awareness. Once they are highlighted by the psychic, they can usually be owned, or at least watched for, by the client. Similarly, an oracle can help one to become aware of unconscious patterns which are operating at the time of a consultation. The material derived from such sources is useful when it is integrated, through reason and common sense, with ongoing understanding of the work in progress. Of course the integrity and expertise of the person accessing such information is extremely important. For instance, I have found that "fortune telling" is rarely helpful over time because it tends to lead a person toward dependency on the fortune teller rather than on deepening one's own internal wisdom. The transpersonal therapist will need to be informed about reliable parapsychological practitioners if this kind of information becomes a part of the growth process.

The therapist will need knowledge, and some experience, of various spiritual practices. As the client enters the stage of spiritual development she will need spiritual practice to foster soul awakening. The soul must be fed, validated, and strengthened, by true "light," or the stream of living Spirit. Within the vessel of vital spiritual practice, higher energies can be received and then stabilized through transpersonal service.

The therapist who understands the client deeply is in the best position to advise him about appropriate practices that can promote spiritual development. Thus, the therapist should be aware of a variety of spiritual practices which can serve people in different ages, stations, religions, and personality types. It is always a great temptation to urge another toward one's own spiritual practice, but the therapist must be as objective as possible in assessing the actual spiritual needs of his client. The client's existing religious beliefs or practices should be honored and worked with to urge him beyond the mechanical repetition of dogma and into a deeper realm of core truth

The knowledge and skill of prayer is often essential. There are conditions in personal life, and of this world, which are clearly beyond our personal will, skill or power. These are the situations which we can bring to prayer, either alone, praying about the client, or with him. Dr. Thomas Parker, author of *Prayer Can Change Your Life*, demonstrated many years ago in the research project described in his book that clients who received prayer together with psychotherapy improved faster and maintained their growth better than counterpart clients who received only psychotherapy. He also discovered how to pray effectively; his book is a fine resource on how to pray for both psychotherapist and clients. Prayer with the client, and/or teaching him how to pray alone, can deepen spiritual development and help to integrate the inner spiritual life with outer life.

Wholistic Awareness

The transpersonal therapist needs to cultivate an awareness of the whole person which can function simultaneously on all channels. By this I mean the ability to follow the client's words, images, body signals, emotional nuances, and energetic emanations, while at the same time attending to one's own internal voices, feelings, body sensations and intuitions. This is no small task, but it is a quality of awareness that has been achieved by many fine therapists. Process Work has recently developed the science of wholistic awareness by differentiating the major parts, or channels, of perception (see especially the work of Arnold Mindell).

Wholeness will be encouraged by the very act of the therapist's respect for it and by his ability to follow the client's whole process. All parts are attended. As the client is seen, heard, felt and believed by the therapist she will more easily respect her own truth and come to accept the validity of her own individuality.

Wholistic awareness also includes attention to nature and the surrounding environment. Client and therapist are together a part of the great flow of the Tao which is reflected to them through synchronous events. Such signals from the environment can highlight and validate the work in progress. I am reminded of a time when both my client and I came to a simultaneous insight that was non-verbal, beyond the ordinary mind, and seemed to originate through the crown chakra. At the moment of our realization, the sun streamed in through the window, lighting up the crown of a Kuan Yin (Goddess of Compassion) figure on the window sill. I had never seen this backlighting effect on her crown, nor have I seen it since. At another time a client was working on the untenable situation (to her) of the traditional male/female relationship. She was saying, "this patriarchal set-up has to change. It should be cracked." At that very moment I heard a sharp cracking sound from the adjacent room that was so alarming that I excused myself to go and see about it. To my amazement I found that a window had cracked right down the middle!

Summary

In this chapter skills, attitudes and practices have been recommended for the transpersonal therapist who wishes to work in a wholistic way toward complete psycho-spiritual development with her clients.

Relationship awareness was described as a way of looking at the work as a team effort, with both therapist and client as constant learners. Explicit relationship skills which can foster trust, intimacy and depth in transformative work were recommended .

Energy awareness was proposed as a necessary skill for attuning with the body and emotions of both client and therapist. Balanced energy, within meridians and chakras, fosters well-being and peacefulness, while imbalanced energy tends to promote an imbalanced working field. It was further emphasized that the energy systems of both therapist and client emanate the qualities of who they are out into the environment; valuable clues about their processes can be read in the field.

Knowledge of the body and its release from obstructive patterns is important in understanding a client's development. The therapist who is aware within her own body also has more resources to access for the work.

Spiritual attunement and information were proposed as necessary components for transpersonal stages of development. It was recommended that both therapist and client align with the soul, when appropriate, so that the work can include spiritual dimensions. Knowledge of various religious and spiritual practices can help the therapist advise the client of spiritual resources that would assist his spiritual development. Prayer and extra-sensory information sources were recommended when appropriate.

Finally, transpersonal therapists were urged to cultivate wholistic awareness that includes simultaneous attention to their own body, emotions and soul and those of their client. Synchronous events were included as meaningful components of the ongoing work.

At the First International Conference on Holistic Health and Medicine in India in 1989, His Holiness the Dalai Lama told us that "Even the Mother Planet itself is asking us to be careful. Even without religion we can manage, but not without love and kindness. As long as the human heart is present in our work, we can reduce negativity." My prayer for this book is that it will promote human love and kindness—for ourselves, our species and our planet.

BIBLIOGRAPHY

The American Heritage Dictionary. New York: Houghton, Mifflin, 1983.

Assagioli, R. *The Act of Will.* New York: Viking Press, 1971.

———— *Psychosynthesis.* New York: Viking Press, 1965.

Aurobindo, Sri. *The Mind of Light.* New York: E.P. Dutton, 1953.

Austin, M. *Acupuncture Therapy.* New York: ASI Publishers, 1972.

Bandler, R., and Grinder, J. *The Structure of Magic, I* (1975) and *II* (1976). Palo Alto: Science and Behavior Books, Inc.

Barker, C.M. *Healing in Depth.* London: Hodder and Stoughton, 1972.

Bennett, H. Z. *Inner Guides, Visions, Dreams & Dr. Einstein: A Field Guide to Inner Resources.* Berkeley, California: Celestial Arts, 1987.

Blofeld, J. *The Secret and Sublime: Taoist Mysteries and Magic.* New York: E.P. Dutton, 1973.

Boorstein, S., ed. *Transpersonal Psychotherapy.* Palo Alto: Science and Behavior Books, Inc., 1980.

Bucke, R. *Cosmic Consciousness.* New York: E.P. Dutton, 1969.

Burr, H. *The Fields of Life.* New York: Ballantine Books, 1973. (out of print)

Capra, F. *A New Vision of Reality and the Nature of Chi.* The Journal of Traditional Acupuncture 7:2 (1975) 110–118.

———— *The Tao of Physics.* New York: Cantom New Age Books, 1975.

Carlson, R., and Shield, B., eds. *Healers on Healing.* Los Angeles: J.P. Tarcher, 1989.

Chitrabhanu, G. *The Psychology of Enlightenment: Meditation on the Seven Energy Centers.* New York: Dodd, Mead and Co., 1979.

Connelly, D. *Traditional Acupuncture: The Law of the Five Elements.* Columbia, Maryland: Center for Traditional Acupuncture, 1979.

Da Free John. *The Knee of Listening.* Clearlake, California: The Dawn Horse Press, 1972.

Dychtwald, K. *Bodymind.* New York: Jove Books, 1977.

Eagles, N. Kala-Huna training. Given in Santa Cruz, California, 1986.

Ferguson, M. *The Brain Revolution.* New York: Taplinger Publishing Co., 1973.

Fiore, E. Lecture delivered at The Association for Past Life Research and Therapy Conference. Oakland, California, October, 1983.

———— *You Have Been Here Before.* New York: Ballantine Books, 1978.

Frankl, V., M.D. *The Doctor and the Soul.* New York: Bantam Books, 1967.

Fritz, R. *The Path of Least Resistance.* New York: Facett, Columbine, 1984.

Gach, M. *Acu-yoga.* Tokyo: Japan Publications, 1981.

Gordon, D. Metaprogram class. Given in Santa Cruz, California, 1980.

Grof, S. *Ancient Wisdom and Modern Science.* Albany: State University of New York Press, 1984.

———— *Beyond the Brain.* Albany: State University of New York Press. 1985.

Gurdjieff. *Views from the Real World.* New York: E.P. Dutton, 1973.

Haas, E. *Staying Healthy With the Seasons.* Millbrae, California: Celestial Arts, 1981.

Hall, M. *The Secret Teachings of All Ages.* Los Angeles: The Philosophical

Research Society, Inc., 1977.

Hammer, L., M.D. *Dragon Rises, Red Bird Flies.* Barrytown, New York: Station Hill Press, 1990.

Harris, T. *I'm O.K.—You're O.K.* New York: Harper & Row, 1967.

Hastings, A.; Fadiman, J.; and Gordon, J. *Health for the Whole Person.* Boulder, Colorado: Westview Press, 1980.

Hendricks, G., and Weinhold, B. *Transpersonal Approaches to Counseling and Psychotherapy.* Denver, Colorado: Love Publishing Co., 1982.

———— Transpersonal Body Therapy Training Seminar. Palo Alto, California, 1984–85.

Hendricks, K. "Transpersonal Body Therapy: A Synthesis of the Theory and Practice." Doctoral dissertation, California Institute of Transpersonal Psychology, 1982.

Jaffe, A. *From the Life and Work of C.G. Jung.* New York: Harper & Row, 1965.

Jampolsky, G. *Love Is Letting Go of Fear.* Berkeley, California: Celestial Arts, 1979.

———— *Teach Only Love.* New York: Bantam Books, 1983.

Janov, A. *The Primal Scream.* New York: Dell Publishing Co., 1971.

Joy, B. *Joy's Way.* Los Angeles: J.P. Tarcher, 1979.

Jung, C.G. *The Archetypes and the Collective Unconscious.* Princeton, New Jersey: Princeton University Press, 1959.

———— *Memories, Dreams and Reflections.* New York: Random House, 1961.

———— *Modern Man In Search of a Soul.* New York: Harcourt Brace and Co., 1933.

———— *Psychological Aspects of the Modern Archetype.* Princeton, New Jersey: Princeton University Press, 1938.

———— *Psychology and Religion: East and West.* New York: Pantheon Books, 1958.

———— *Symbols of Transformation.* Princeton, New Jersey: Princeton University Press, 1967.

Kaptchuk, T. *The Web That Has No Weaver: Understanding Chinese Medicine.* New York: Congdon and Weed, 1983.

Keleman, S. *Your Body Speaks Its Mind: The Bio-energetic Way to Greater Emotional and Sexual Satisfaction.* New York: Simon and Schuster, 1975.

Kronemeyer, R. "Syntonic Therapy: A Total Approach to the Treatment of Mental and Emotional Disturbances." *Psychotherapy: Theory, Research and Practice* 14:3 (1977) 249–253.

Krystal, P. *Cutting More Ties That Bind.* Longmeade, Shaftsbury, Dorset, England: Element Books, 1990.

Kubie, L. "The Neurotic Process as the Focus of Physiological and Psychoanalytic Research." *The Journal of Mental Science* 104 (1958) 123–134.

Kübler-Ross, E. *Death: The Final Stage of Growth.* Englewood Cliffs, New Jersey: Prentice Hall, 1975.

Kurtz, R., and Prestera, H. *The Body Reveals.* New York: Harper & Row, 1976.

Lao Tsu. *Tao Te Ching.* Trans. by Fia Fu Feng and Jane English. New York: Random House, 1972.

Lawson-Wood, D., and Lawson-Wood, J. *Five Elements of Acupuncture and Chinese Massage*. Rustington, England: Health Science Press, 1965.

Leadbeater, C.W. *The Chakras*. Wheaton, Illinois: Theosophical Publishing House, 1927.

Leonard, G. *The Silent Pulse*. New York: Bantam Books, 1981.

Leung, K. *Chinese Medical Philosophy and Principles of Diagnosis*. Los Angeles: The North American College of Acupuncture, 1971.

Lowen, A. *Bioenergetics*. Middlesex, England: Penguin Books, 1975.

——— *The Language of the Body*. New York: Collier Books, 1958.

MacNutt, F. *Healing*. New York: Ave Marie Press, 1974.

Mann, W. *Orgone, Reich and Eros*. New York: Simon and Schuster, 1973.

Maslow, A. *The Farther Reaches of Human Nature*. New York: The Viking Press, 1971.

Matsumoto, K., and Birch, S. *Five Elements and Ten Stems*. Brookline, Maryland: Paradigm Publications, 1983.

Merrell-Wolff, F. *Pathways Through Space*. New York: Julian Press, 1973.

Miller, A. *The Drama of Being a Child*. London: Virago Press Limited, 1987.

Mindell, A. *Dreambody: The Body's Role in Revealing the Self*. Santa Monica, California: Sigo Press, 1982.

——— *River's Way*. London: Routledge & Kegan Paul, 1985.

———*Working With the Dreaming Body*. London: Routledge & Kegan Paul, 1985.

Monroe, R. *Journeys Out of the Body*. Garden City, New Jersey: Doubleday , 1971.

Mookerjee, A. *Kundalini: The Inner Energy*. New York: Destiny Books, 1982.

Montgomery, R. *Born To Heal*. New York: Popular Library, 1976.

Moss, R. *The I That Is We*. Millbrae, California: Celestial Arts, 1981.

Montoyama, H. *Theories of the Chakras*. Wheaton, Illinois: Theosophical Publishing House, 1981.

——— and Frown, R. *Science and the Evolution of Consciousness*. Brookline, Mass: Autumn Press, 1978.

Murray, D. *A History of Western Psychology*. Englewood Cliffs, New Jersey: Prentice Hall, 1983.

Ni, Hua-Ching. *8000 Years of Wisdon: Conversations with Taoist Master Ni, Hua-Ching*. Malibu, California: The Shrine of the Eternal Breath, 1983.

——— *Tao: The Subtle Universal Law and the Integral Way of Life*. Los Angeles: College of Tao and Traditional Chinese Healing, 1979.

——— *The Taoist Inner View of the Universe and the Immortal Realm*. Malibu, California: The Shrine of the Eternal Breath, 1979.

Nordenstrom, B. *Biologically Closed Electric Circuits: Clinical, Experimental, and Theoretical Evidence for an Additional Circulatory System*. Stockholm, Sweden: Self-published, 1983.

O'Connor, J., and Bensky, D., trans. *Acupuncture: A Comprehensive Text*. Chicago: Eastland Press for Shanghai College of Traditional Medicine, 1981.

Omura, Y. *Acupuncture Medicine: Its Historical and Clinical Background*. Tokyo:

Japan Publications, 1982.

Ouspensky, P. *The Psychology of Man's Possible Evolution*. London: Hedgehog Press, 1950.

Painter, J. W. *Deep Bodywork and Personal Development*. Mill Valley, California: Self-published, 1984.

Parker, W. *Prayer Can Change Your Life*. New York: Cornerstone Library, 1957.

――― *Prayer Therapy*. Newport Beach, California: Self-published, 1969.

Penfield, W. *The Mystery of the Mind*. Princeton, New Jersey: Princeton University Press, 1975.

Radha, S. *Kundalini Yoga for the West*. Spokane, Washington: Timeless Books, 1978.

Raheem, A. *Process Acupressure*. Santa Cruz, California: Self-published, 1990.

Rama, S.; Ballentine, R., M.D.; and Ajaya, S. *Yoga and Psychotherapy: The Evolution of Consciousness*. Honesdale, Pennsylvania: Himalayan International Institute, 1976.

Reich, W. *Character Analysis*. New York: Farrar, Straus & Giroux, 1949.

Rolf, I. *Structural Integration: The Recreation of the Balanced Human Body*. New York: Viking Press, 1977.

Rosenberg, J.L. *Body, Self and Soul: Sustaining Integration*. Atlanta, Georgia: Humanics Limited, 1985.

Roshi, K., and Phillamy, D. *The Book of Life*. Mt. Shasta, California: Shasta Abbey Press, 1979.

Sanford, A. *The Healing Gifts of the Spirit*. Philadelphia: Trumpet Books, 1966.

Schwarz, J. *Human Energy Systems*. New York: E.P. Dutton, 1980.

――― *The Path of Action*. New York: E.P. Dutton, 1977.

――― *Voluntary Controls*. New York: E.P. Dutton, 1978.

Sheldon, W.; Stevens, S.; and Tucker, W. *The Varieties of Human Physique*. New York: Harper & Row, 1940.

Sheldrake, R. *A New Science of Life*. Los Angeles: J.P. Tarcher, 1981.

Singer, J. *Boundaries of the Soul*. Garden City, New Jersey: Anchor Books, 1972.

――― *Energies of Love: Sexuality Re-visioned*. Garden City, New Jersey: Doubleday Books, 1983.

Smith, F., M.D. *Inner Bridges: A Guide to Energy Movement and Body Structure*. Atlanta, Georgia: Humanics New Age, 1986.

Stapleton, R. *The Experience of Inner Healing*. Waco, Texas: Word Books, 1977.

Stone, H. *Embracing Heaven and Earth*. Marina del Rey, California: DeVorss & Co., 1985.

Stone, H., and Winkelman, S. *Voice Dialogue: A Tool for Transformation*. Los Angeles: Delos Books, 1977.

Sumohadiwidjojo, M. *Susila Budhi Dharma*. London: Subud Publications International, 1975.

Tart, C. *Altered States of Consciousness*. New York: John Wiley and Sons, 1969.

Teeguarden, I. *Acupressure Way of Health: Jin Shin Do*. Tokyo: Japan Publications, 1978.

――― *The Body Mandala*. Idyllwild, California: Jin Shin Do Foundation, 1982.

―――― *The Joy of Feeling: Bodymind Acupressure*. Tokyo: Japan Publications, 1986.

Tobin, B. *Space-time and Beyond*. New York: E.P. Dutton, 1975.

Toor, A. Personal conversation, 1983.

Upledger, J., M.D. *Somato-Emotional Release*. Palm Beach Gardens, Florida: U.I. Publishing, 1990

Veith, I. *The Yellow Emperor's Classic of Internal Medicine*. Berkeley: University of California Press, 1949.

Walker, B. *Masks of the Soul*. Wellingborough, Northamptonshire, England: The Aquarian Press, 1981.

Walsh, R., and Vaughan, F., eds. *Beyond Ego: Transpersonal Dimensions in Psychology*. Los Angeles: J. P. Tarcher, 1980.

Watts, A. *Tao: The Watercourse Way*. New York: Pantheon Books, 1975.

Weatherhead, A. *Psychology, Religion and Healing*. New York: Abingdon-Cokesbury Press, 1951.

Westlake, A. *The Pattern of Health*. Boulder, Colorado: Shambhala Press, 1973.

White Eagle. *The Path of the Soul*. Hampshire, England: White Eagle Publishing Trust, 1980.

Wilber, K. *The Atman Project*. Wheaton, Illinois: Theosophical Publishing House, 1980.

―――― *The Holographic Paradigm*. Boulder, Colorado: Shambhala Press, 1982.

Wilhelm, R. *The Secret of the Golden Flower*. New York: Harcourt Brace Jovanovich, 1962.

Williston, F., and Johnstone, J. *Soul Search*. Wellingborough, Northamptonshire, England: Turnstone Publishers, 1983.

Wurmbrand, R. *In God's Underground*. Glendale, California: Diane Books Publishing Co., 1968.

Yogananda, P. *Autobiography of a Yogi*. Los Angeles: Self-Realization Fellowship, 1946.

Zukav, G. *The Dancing Wu Li Masters*. New York: Bantam Books, 1980.

INDEX

Personal Power Cards   by Barbara Gress

Personal Power Cards is a simple, easy to use set of flash cards for emotional wellness. Each set includes 55 cards, a carrying pouch, and an 80 page book. The Cards help retrain your feelings to be positive and healthy. Their combination of colors, shapes, and words allows positive thoughts to penetrate deep into your subconscious, "programming" your emotions for health.

"In the twenty years I have been using color and mind imagery with patients, I have never seen any approach have such a great benefit on self-discipline and self-esteem. " —Richard Shames, M.D., Family Practitioner and author of *Healing with Mind Power*

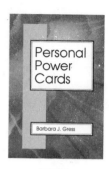

$18.95

Intuition Workout   by Nancy Rosanoff

This practical training manual teaches simple techniques to access our deepest sources of inner knowing in any situation.

The author, one of America's outstanding corporate trainers, shows that intuition, like a muscle, is strengthened by training. She outlines dozens of case histories and step-by-step exercises proven effective even with "non-intuitive" people.

"A workout in cultivating our inner resources and building self-confidence. Once you know how to do it, you can adapt the techniques to any situation."
—New York Daily News

Available as a book or audio tape.
Also sold as a set for a $3 discount.

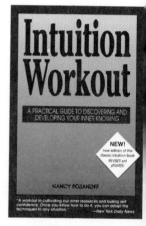

$10.95 book/$9.95 tape

Your Body Believes Every Word You Say   by Barbara Levine

This is the first book to describe the language of the link between mind and body. Barbara Levine's fifteen-year battle with a huge brain tumor led her to trace common phrases like "that breaks my heart" and "it's a pain in the butt" back to the underlying beliefs on which they are based and the symptoms they cause. She lists hundreds of common examples of words we use unconsciously every day, and shows how these "seedthoughts" can set us up for illness.

"Barbara Levine's journey is one of courage and growth. We can all learn from her experience. She shows us what we are capable of an how to achieve our full healing potential."
—Bernie Siegel, M.D.

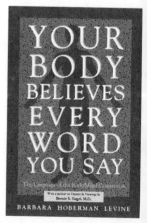

$11.95

The Heart of the Healer
Edited by Dawson Church & Dr. Alan Sherr

A collection of outstanding figures on the leading edge of conventional and holistic medicine, including Bernie Siegel, Norman Cousins and Prince Charles, draw on their deepest personal experiences to explore how we get in touch with the essence of wellness. This classic has been called "Exceptional" —*SSC Booknews*; "Thought-provoking" —*Publisher's Weekly*; "Profound...provocative" —*Ram Dass*.

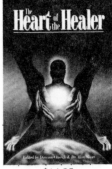

$14.95

Voice Power
by Dr. Joan Kenley

The sound of your voice can have more than five times the impact of the words you say. *Voice Power* shows you how to draw on the resources of your whole body to release your natural voice—the voice that is truly and fully you. It shows you how to integrate the deepest roots of your personality, your vitality and your sexuality, to project charisma and confidence.

"...a fun read as well as a very practical, thorough book." —*Network Magazine*

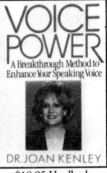

$18.95 Hardback

Love is a Secret
by Andrew Vidich

What is God's love and how do we experience it. Drawing on the words of saints and scholars from a rich variety of religious traditions, from Taoism to Christianity, from Sufism to Judaism, this book illuminates the psychology of humankind's deepest spiritual experiences.

"In a world yearning to find its unity and connectedness, this book invokes for all to hear, 'Love has only a beginning, my friend; it has no ending.' "
—*Dr Arthur Stein, Professor Peace Studies, Univ. of R.I.*

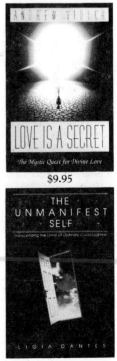

$9.95

The Unmanifest Self
by Ligia Dantes

This book, like a warm, gentle friend, guides us toward an experience of self-transformation that is quite different from our usual waking consciousness, that is vastly more than an improved version of the old self. *The Unmanifest Self* teaches us the art of *objective self-observation*, a powerful tool to separate the essential truth of who we are from the labyrinth of thoughts and emotions in which we are often caught.

"...beautiful and inspiring." —*Willis Harmon*

$9.95

Order Form

(Please print legibly)　　　　　　　　Date ————————

Name ——————————————————————————————

Address ——————————————————————————————

City ————————————————— State ——— Zip ——————————

Phone ——————————————————————————————

Please send a catalog to my friend:

Name ——————————————————————————————

Address ——————————————————————————————

City ————————————————— State ——— Zip ——————————

Quantity Discounts!

$2 off if you order 2 items
$3 off if you order 3 items
$4 off if you order 4 items, etc...

Item	Qty.	Price	Amount
Personal Power Cards		$18.95	
Intuition Workout (book)		$10.95	
Intuition Workout (tape)		$9.95	
Your Body Believes Every Word You Say		$11.95	
The Heart of the Healer		$14.95	
Voice Power (hardback book)		$18.95	
Love is a Secret		$9.95	
The Unmanifest Self		$9.95	
		Subtotal	
		Quantity Discount	
	Calif. res. add 8.25% sales tax		
		Shipping	
		Grand Total	

Add for shipping:
Domestic　$3.00 for first item, 50¢ each additional item
Canada/Mexico: One and one half domestic rates
Foreign: Double domestic rates

Check type of payment:

☐ Check or money order enclosed

☐ VISA　　☐ MasterCard

Acct. # ——————————————————

Exp. Date ——————————————————

Signature ——————————————————

Send order to:
Aslan Publishing
PO Box 108
Lower Lake, CA 95457

or call to order:
(707) 995-3906
(800) 275-2606

SR

Order Form

(Please print legibly)

Date _____

Name _____

Address _____

City _____ State _____ Zip _____

Phone _____

Please send a catalog to my friend:

Name _____

Address _____

City _____ State _____ Zip _____

Quantity Discounts!

$2 off if you order 2 items
$3 off if you order 3 items
$4 off if you order 4 items, etc...

Item	Qty.	Price	Amount
Personal Power Cards		$18.95	
Intuition Workout (book)		$10.95	
Intuition Workout (tape)		$9.95	
Your Body Believes Every Word You Say		$11.95	
The Heart of the Healer		$14.95	
Voice Power (hardback book)		$18.95	
Love is a Secret		$9.95	
The Unmanifest Self		$9.95	
		Subtotal	
		Quantity Discount	
	Calif. res. add 8.25% sales tax		
		Shipping	
		Grand Total	

Add for shipping:
Domestic $3.00 for first item, 50¢ each additional item
Canada/Mexico: One and one half domestic rates
Foreign: Double domestic rates

Check type of payment:

☐ Check or money order enclosed

☐ VISA   ☐ MasterCard

Acct. # _____

Exp. Date _____

Signature _____

Send order to:
Asian Publishing
PO Box 108
Lower Lake, CA 95457

or call to order:
(707) 995-3906
(800) 275-2606

SR